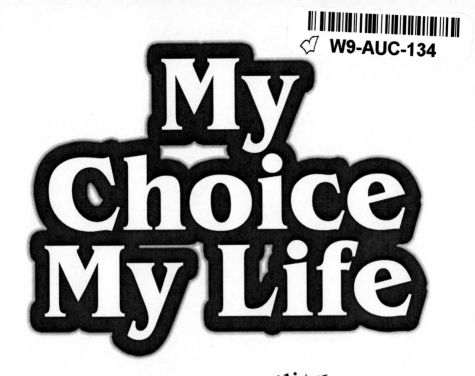

My Choice My Life

Realizing Your Ability

to Create Balance in Life

Jay M. Greenfeld, Ph.D.

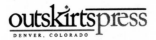

outskirtspress

DENVER, COLORADO

ACKNOWLEDGMENTS

To my parents: Roz and Marty Greenfeld have been an instrumental part of my life, giving me the roots to grow strong and the wings to fly high. I cannot thank them enough for their continued support, challenge, encouragement, and teaching me what it means to respect, trust, and be honest with myself and each and every person I interact with. If I can one day be half the parental figure they exemplify, I know my children will succeed. I cannot say enough about how much I appreciate all the little things they have done and continue to do that help shape me as a person. Therefore, Mom and Dad, with all my love I say quite simply – THANK YOU.

To my uncle, Keevin Bernstein: Without him the idea of this book never would have happened. I used to regularly meet him on Sunday mornings for an exercise and breakfast date. We would engage in numerous topics, ranging from children, work, and life to thoughts and experiences. He dropped me off one day and jokingly said: "You should really write a book on your thoughts and ideas." Well, Keev, the idea never left my mind and whether you were kidding or not, here it is. Your continued support for my ideas, reflections, and creativity is and has always been cherished– THANK YOU.

To Sarah L. Shell: She helped me to understand that I can be successful with any idea, even if it means taking a chance. We had many discussions about what I wanted to include in this book and she asked me, "What is preventing that from happening? Make it happen!" She continuously communicates that it is okay to be unique and spontaneous without settling for mediocrity. Sarah, your devotion to helping me articulate the ideas I wanted to communicate throughout the book is something I am so grateful for. Therefore, I can easily and enthusiastically say: THANK YOU.

The Reference Section. The reference section is located at the back of the book and is intended to be an added tool for the reader. There are a number of terms and concepts that I will mention throughout the book which I did not create myself; nor am I claiming to. Thus, it is essential that proper credit is given to the individuals who helped create these terms and concepts, and select individuals who helped further the research in the various areas. There are a variety of ways to attribute proper credit and recognition to the research completed in a given area. I have chosen a method that allows for the book to flow without the content and layout feeling like an academic textbook or a historical reflection on healthy living.

Each time a term is introduced and a small number appears above the word or phrase, the proper association can be found in the reference section. The selected citations within each number are listed in ascending chronological order. The author(s) who originally developed or helped create the idea is listed, followed by who further added to the research in subsequent years within affiliated fields of study. The purpose is to provide resources and citations for many terms I emphasize, and moreover, to attribute proper credit to the individuals who helped create and enhance the literature on topics that can lead to balancing life. It is essential to acknowledge those who initiated the terms, theories, and concepts that have become familiar in our language of healthy living.

"To laugh often and much, to win the respect of intelligent people and the affection of children, to earn the appreciation of honest critics and endure the betrayal of false friends, to appreciate beauty, to find the best in others, to leave the world a bit better, whether by a healthy child, a garden patch... to know even one life has breathed easier because you have lived. This is to have succeeded."
~Ralph Waldo Emerson

TABLE OF CONTENTS

CHAPTER 1   Balancing Your Game Board of Life ... 1

CHAPTER 2   Putting Your Mental Skills to the Test.. 19

CHAPTER 3   Physical Balance – With More Than
Just Two Feet on the Ground 31

CHAPTER 4   Emotional and Mental Balance –
Working With the Inside
for the Best Outside 43

CHAPTER 5   Social Balance – Ties Within
the Core of the Family Tree 63

CHAPTER 6   Social Balance – Extending out
to the Branches of the Tree 81

CHAPTER 7   It's a Jungle out There: The
Powerful Influence of Friendships 89

CHAPTER 8   Dating...Winning a Game
You Choose to Play 105

CHAPTER 9   Social Balance: The Local Street
                 Pharmacy of Social Circles 119

CHAPTER 10   The Twenties and Far Beyond...
                 Mentally and Chronologically 127

CHAPTER 11   Academic and Professional
                 Balance – Anticipation and
                 Preparation for Success 153

CHAPTER 12   Unnecessary Roughness:
                 Embracing Chronic Illness 169

CHAPTER 13   Making the Impossible...Possible 185

Appendix A   Progressive Muscle Relaxation 199

Appendix B   Exercise Plan 203

Appendix C   Meal Plan.. 209

Appendix D   The Graduate School
                 Application Process 215

Appendix E   Mastering Your Interviews 225

References 231

PREFACE

I have had a long-standing passion for integrating balance into my life as well as the lives of others. The current book is not another self-help book promising that if you read it from cover to cover you will be in control of everything you do in your life and your whole world will be wonderful, like a picture of rainbows, flowers, and waterfalls. Instead, the purpose of this book is to give you insight into how you think about yourself and the choices you make. Balancing your life can be seen in many different ways. The focus of the current book is to stress the how, why, and when balance can happen throughout your teens, twenties, and beyond.

The intended audience is not age-specific, but directed more to individuals at various life stages, including both parents *and* children. If you are in high school, college, or graduate school, or if you are a young professional, this book is here to help you understand and practice balance in your life. If you have or will have children in the aforementioned life stages, this book is intended to help you better understand what they may experience, may be experiencing, or have already experienced, to open all lines of communication with them and yourself.

I discuss four areas of life that I feel are the cornerstones to balanced healthy living: physical, emotional, social, and professional. We often say "If only I had thought about it before I did something, I would have been better off." The key to balancing parts of your life is acknowledging that you can think about it, which can change your actions.

We often regret certain behaviors or actions that we cannot retract. However, the advantage to thinking first before acting is that it allows you to retract without the repercussions of your thoughts affecting someone else. You can always go back on your thoughts, but not your actions. It is my belief that the balance helps you understand that your thoughts are within your control, and what you choose to do with those thoughts can help govern your actions. How and what each of the four elements can look like will be outlined; offering suggestions, provoking thought, and creating awareness to how balanced healthy living is feasible.

Physical balance emphasizes how it is possible to engage in regular exercise, routine healthy eating, and weight control. Emotional balance highlights how you can take control of your thoughts, feelings, and the resulting behaviors. The main point to understand is that you can be in check with your emotions and accept that you will have distress in your life. How well-balanced you are emotionally stems from the choices you make. The book will attempt to capture how you can make room in your life to think about your thoughts and take responsibility for your choices to clarify how you feel. Social balance lies in a number of different areas: your family, your friends, your social activities, and many more. The belief is that there are going to be a number of aspects that help define your social life. The hope is that you can separate each of them to ensure you have time, heart, and energy to devote to all aspects of your social world.

Finally, there is the challenge of professional balance. How can you have enough hours of work and/or school and still somehow make time for everything else in your life? Well, I will tell you it is possible if you want it to be. We all have a million things to do during one school or work day. The key is to see how the puzzle pieces of each day all fit together without going to bed when the sun rises.

The terminology throughout the book is intended to apply to a diverse audience. There are a variety of ways to present information that account for all readers regardless of the color of their skin, preference in dating and life partners, religious practices, age, and the amount of money, assets, and education they may have. I have chosen to take a wide-ranging perspective in the hope of remaining sensitive to all of the above and more. Everyone's family dynamics and life story will look different. It is important to be aware of the differences within and between us when expressing ideas of what balance will look like for each person.

You may not use all the ideas in this book. I do not attempt to give you life's answers. Instead, I offer you hints, tools, techniques, and suggestions. The key for you is to take what you want from each page and apply it to your life, your world, and on your time. I strongly suggest you do not rush through the material. It may be information you have thought about before, but felt it did not apply directly to you. I attempt to personalize the information in a way that will help reveal you can make small changes in your life and the lives of others. The small changes we can make may help create a healthy balance between our head, heart, and body. It may be most helpful to read one chapter at a time, reflect on it, and implement the techniques from that chapter before you move to the next one.

To make things easy and most helpful, I have included pages at the end of each chapter and at the back of the book for you to write reflective thoughts or personal reactions to the content you read. The space is provided for you to process exactly what you are thinking at certain moments in time related to you and your life. So, as you go through the pages, feel free to write down your favorite quotes, page numbers, and tools that you want to remember. After each chapter, go to the notes page or the back of the book and write down the messages you want to take from it. Feel free to circle, underline, and highlight anything that triggers a thought in your mind as you read. Instead of thinking "I wish I could remember that line." Write it down so you will remember it. Everyone will pick different items to attend to. The key is: This is your book, and you have the choice to write down what is most important to you.

The main idea is that this book is to be a helpful tool that you can use at various stages in your life. The problem is that, whether we realize it or not, we re-evaluate our lives every four years (e.g., after elementary school, high school, college, professional degrees, etc.). However, very rarely do we truly remember what we were thinking and feeling during those times. Thus, I say: Write down your thoughts, feelings, and goals throughout the book and after each chapter. In a few years, return to the book and reread the notes you have written. How are they different? How are they the same? What do you want to change?

I want to help you understand that you have the power to take charge of your life. Each day that you wake up, you are given the opportunity to roll the dice. You *can* choose how to live your life every time the sun rises. Good things and bad things will happen. You *can* enjoy your time in a balanced, purposeful, determined, and successful way. Pay close attention to each moment and each page that you read in the following chapters. Whether you choose to read this on the subway, the trains, at the park, in your home, or on the plane, do not rush. There are no grades or salary bonuses for reading this. The book is for your enjoyment, your growth, and your benefit.

CHAPTER 1
Balancing Your
Game Board of Life

"Our lives are not determined by what happens to us but by how we react to what happens, not by what life brings to us, but by the attitude we bring to life. A positive attitude causes a chain reaction of positive thoughts, events, and outcomes. It is a catalyst, a spark that creates extraordinary results."
~Anonymous

Creating a balance in life is not one of the easiest tasks. How do we do it, what is involved, and what aspects do we need to include to balance our lives? It seems as though in my experience working and interacting with many children, adolescents, college students, and young professionals, (and often their parents), the key to balance in life is supported by four dimensions. The four dimensions include: physical, emotional and mental, social, and academic or professional.

We live in a fast-paced, competitive world where more money goes to the development of professional sports arenas than efforts to decrease a high obesity rate and better our education system. We learn the concept of competition early in life, which remains with us throughout the passage of time. The fast-paced society we live in forces us to pay too much attention to some aspects of life, and too little to others. We have too little time to consider our thoughts and feelings and what we truly want from life. Most of us are concerned with finding the ability to balance everything life throws at us and still end up on our feet at the end of the day. Is it possible to balance everything we have in our lives? And if so, how? I truly believe it is possible.

I perceive that life is like a Monopoly® board. The actual word monopoly can be synonymous with words like dictatorship, domination, power, and rule over other individuals. However, I am interested in drawing a parallel between the strategy of the board game and how we manage our thoughts, feelings, and actions to navigate our lives. I believe that every single piece or idea of that board game can be compared to life. The same route and strategies you use to succeed in Monopoly®, the board game, you can use in life to balance the four major aspects mentioned above. The hope in life is to have full ownership of the places, things, and spaces on the metaphorical game board. The same can be said for life. You want to make every attempt to have ownership and/or control of the whole board of your life, and not let others control your fate.

Anyone who has spent time playing Monopoly® knows the best part about the game is it can go on until you say I have had enough! The hope, though, is that you have put everything you can into the game before calling it quits. Before I even get into the spaces on the board itself, I want to explain how the pieces in the box fit with the metaphor. Essentially, you have the option to pick from one of twelve pieces or images to represent who you are: the car, the hat, the thimble, the dog, etc. You can choose only one, and you focus on that one for the whole game. My belief is that each of those pieces represents a stage in your life. Therefore, you play the game once with those pieces, and at the next stage in your life you pick another piece and play again.

For example, at the age of twelve to fifteen you choose the hat and you move around the board as the hat. Then as you are entering high school, you say to yourself, "Okay, who do I want to be for the next four years?" and you pick the car. Then you chose the dog for the stage of college years. The actual piece is irrelevant. What is important is that you choose an image and circle the board until that stage in life is complete, at least for you.

Then we move on to the money. Monopoly® money is divided into seven increments (e.g., 1, 5, 10, 20, 50, 100, and 500). The money is analogous to time, how much you have and how much you want to invest in certain things. You have to realize we all start with the same amount of money in the game, better known as time. We differ in how and where we choose to invest it. For example, one person could be twenty-three and choose to invest most of their time seeking a significant other or attending to a drug habit. Consequently, this person will not have as much time (money) available to focus on work or maintain regular exercise. The idea is that we all make the choice every time we pick up the dice to roll.

Next is the deck of cards, otherwise known as the properties that are available to purchase. In life we all have the option to invest in certain properties more than others. The properties resemble aspects of life in which we choose to take ownership. More detail as to what each set of properties, railroads, and utilities applies to will be discussed later. However, for now just be aware of what the properties mean in life. The properties are what you buy in the game. You make the conscious choice to either put down a certain amount of money to guarantee you own that property, because without hesitation you know you want control over that. You want to hope you have control over how you spend your time.

Finally the last game piece(s): the hotels and houses. These little structures represent permanence, a stronghold over certain aspects of your life. For example, it is not enough to just own the property, because at any given time, if you are out of resources or not careful with your choices, you could lose it. If you do not establish yourself on that property, anyone can take it from you at any time.

Now for the game board itself. We move around

from square to square trying to accomplish as much as we can in each step. We move around the board until we have hopefully monopolized our life at a certain stage. There are four rows on the board running along each side. The idea is that each side represents a different aspect of balancing life: physical balance, mental and emotional balance, social balance, and academic or professional balance. In the actual Monopoly® game itself, as you move around the board, the properties increase in value, and become more difficult to obtain. The key is to know what is worth the most to you at your present stage in life.

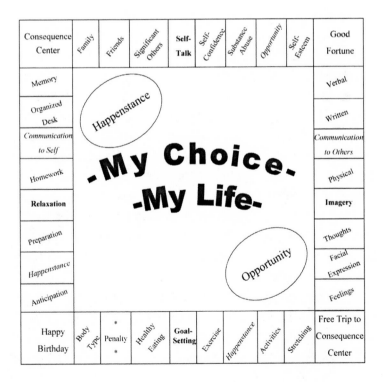

Therefore, the first time you play the game, you begin with the properties that are easiest to obtain. Not much effort is required to take ownership of them. For some people the social aspect may be first; academic success or physical development may be the most difficult and therefore is the last row. For others, the academic aspect may be the easiest and school work or professional work may come naturally. Therefore, the first row is academic or professional balance. However, finding companionship and a strong group of friends is more difficult and thus would be the last row. Whichever row you begin with — social, academic or professional, physical, or mental and emotional — the idea is that you yourself will know what is easiest to obtain.

As you move along, you pass some unusual squares. First are the *Railroads*. The railroads are not properties you have to own, but if you can control all four of them you know you will gain easily, as they are passed by often. Therefore, the railroads are equivalent to the mental skills of Self-talk[1], Relaxation[2], Imagery[3], and Goal-setting.[4] It is not crucial that you have all of these under control, but it can definitely help long-term. These skills can act as preventive measures, creating more awareness of your feelings and accomplishments.

The next unusual squares are the utilities, *Water* and *Electricity*. Those two aspects are not essential to own, and you do not gain very much by having them individually, but if you have both of them you may be far better off. Thus, the utilities represent two types of communication, which include: (1) communication with yourself, making sure you are constantly in-check with yourself and who is most important to you, and (2) communication with others.[5] Do not be afraid to communicate the same thoughts to others that you do to yourself, as it can enhance your development and any relationship.[6] Continuously communicating with yourself about how you are feeling and what you are thinking, as well as checking in with what others are thinking, may help provide insight into your world.

The next squares include *Opportunity (Community Chest)* and *Happenstance*[7] *(Chance)*. You may be proceeding through life on a specific path with certain ideas in your head as to where you want to go or where you want to be at a certain age, but you have to factor in happenstance. Happenstance includes the things in life that happen because of coincidence, luck, or chance.[7] We can attempt to control as much as we want in our lives, but it is essential to factor in chance and life working in mysterious ways sometimes. Contrary to what some believe, we cannot plan everything in life, and we must be prepared for chance. As you get closer to those squares, you know in the back of your mind that there is a possibility you may land on opportunity or happenstance and thus have to embrace life's uncertainties. When you land on those squares and you are asked to pick up a card from the center of the board, you never know what will be on the other side. It is not so much what the card says, but more so how you react to it that can help contribute to balance.

Things can and will happen that are out of your control (e.g., a death in the family, a pay raise at work, a cancelled class at school, a significant other cheating on you, or an injury). Whether good things or bad things happen, you know that the game does not stop. When you play Monopoly® and pick up one of those little cards with some unlucky news, the game does not end, and you do not quit. You attempt to grow from the consequences or gain from the luxuries, and carry on. Life delivers some punches, but if you are ready for them and know how to handle them, you have a great chance of bouncing back.

Moving along, you pass two squares that result in you paying taxes on two separate occasions: property and luxury. Those two squares are simply saying that good fortune and a strong balance will come at a price. You have to keep reminding yourself that just because you have ownership of certain aspects, it is not a free ride from there. You have to maintain what you have, and therefore pay the taxes to ensure that others have similar opportunities later in life. The taxes emerge in the form of effort. Not everything will come easy to you, and it will require your effort and responsibility to maintain your balance.

The four corners of the board represent different elements of life. The first corner you pass is the *Jail*. No, that does not mean everyone goes to jail, but the square resembles a cool-down period that gives you time to consider your actions. The jail square is more like a Consequence Center. You have tried to skip a step in life, you have tried to cut a corner — you may get away with it the first few times, but eventually you will get caught. Thus, go to jail and take a breather, reflect upon how you got there, and think about what you will do to avoid returning.

The Good Fortune square (*Free Parking*) is a sweet reminder that every so often good fortunes come to those who wait and those who keep trying. The good fortunes are the once-in-a-lifetime joys that provide a sense of satisfaction for your efforts. That does not mean you will win the lottery and you will have millions of dollars. However, you may get accepted into graduate school, receive a promotion at work, obtain your driver's license, win a gold medal in the Olympics, make your Little League squad, make the high school basketball team, score high on your LSAT or MCAT – or, dare I say it, experience the joy of finding your life partner.

Whatever the case is, good fortune does not happen often and is very exciting when it does. Landing on this square is far greater than any opportunity and happenstance card you may receive. The Good Fortune square is something you are beyond ecstatic to receive and will always enjoy, as it is a rare occurrence.

The Free Trip to Consequence Center (*Go to Jail*) square is quite obvious. Simply being caught in the act of trying to cut too many corners earns you a free trip to the Consequence Center. The time spent in the center is for you to pay attention to why taking the easy way out in achieving your dreams may not be best. Life is not about cutting corners; it is about experiencing everything to earn your success. If you cut too many corners, it will catch up with you at some point. That is not saying that you cannot cut corners, as many people do, but sooner or later you will have to put the work in to it.

Lastly, every time you pass the "Happy Birthday"

(GO) square you collect two hundred dollars. The square where it all began is comparable to having a birthday. You spend so much time on each square, investing a lot of effort and energy in mastering each aspect. By the time you get to the GO square, it is usually a birthday, anniversary, or any such milestone. The square is to act as a simple reminder to remember where you came from and provide you with an opportunity to reflect on your year that passed.

We will move around the board and use an example of how life plays out in a simple round of Monopoly®. Each side has two sets of properties on it. Therefore, within each of the four cornerstones of balance in life they are divided into two, and within the two each one is divided into a set of either two or a set of three. For example, if your first side is academic or professional success, meaning you have a natural ability to succeed in both school and work life with little effort, that type of material comes naturally to you. It is important to know that everyone's game board will look different. Some include more opportunity, better luck, or more struggle. So, the number of squares will vary from person to person, but the elements that create balance (*properties*) will always look the same.

Within academic or professional success you have two categories balancing work. The first is life outside of work (the first two properties), ensuring everything is ready for the next day — or if it is school, making sure all your homework is done so you are not going to bed anxious, worried, and unprepared. The first set of academic or professional success begins with anticipation and preparation. The second set of properties is divided into three, which is balancing your work or school life at work or while at school. That would mean making sure you are well-prepared for each class, paying attention to each task, doing your homework, and working at an organized desk without papers in all directions. That may also include retaining all the information you need to prepare for either when you get home, when you have a test, or the next time this scenario presents itself at work and/or school. Therefore, the next time you are faced with the same scenario(s), you are ready and not overwhelmed.

The main idea is to be prepared. Once you are completely prepared, managing everything you need to in and out of work — and, most importantly, you are ready for any task put forth in front of you — it is time to roll the dice and move on. Of course, over and above it all you want to have full control and start building "*houses* and *hotels*" on those properties. You want to make sure you are not using your family time, spare time, or leisure time to attain this level of balance. Last, but not least, you may be ready for anything, but be prepared for landing on "Happenstance" or visiting the Consequence Center, as those same squares are within that first lap of the board.

Nevertheless, you are happy with the way you have balanced your work life in and out of the office or school. Now roll again and round the corner, either hitting or missing the "Consequence Center" square. From the Consequence Center square you move on to the next aspect of balance: social balance. Social balance is divided into two categories with three properties in each: family, friends, and significant others are in one set. The second set includes personal thoughts that enhance and balance your socialization, and your decisions in the three areas.

The second set includes three areas (properties) that have less to do with interaction and more to do with your inner social drive, self-esteem[27], self-confidence, and substance use and/or abuse. Each of these processes involves choices you can make on your own, independent of others. The first set of social properties requires other people to confirm that you have balanced your family, friends, and significant others. The second set of social properties involves your thoughts and personal beliefs regarding what can decrease, maintain, or enhance your social world. Again, you will pass the Opportunity square, so be prepared for it. Be prepared that it is not all smooth sailing just because you land where you do. Remember you are rolling the dice continuously until you are as close as you can be to being as completely balanced in all four aspects as you choose to be.

So you roll again and move into the next row of properties: mental or emotional balance. These two sets of properties again have three within each. The first set of three are all coded under forms of expression: verbal[15], physical,[16] and written.[17] The idea here is that to be certain you are balancing your emotions and expressing them effectively you will use all three outlets. Keep in mind that some people do not work well with written expression and therefore would probably not buy into the property or would buy it for the set, but might not build on it.

The second set of mental or emotional balance is

the nonverbal expression[8] of your inner thoughts and feelings, which includes: facial expression (how often do you smile?), thoughts (are you too stressed, or anxious so often that you become short of breath?), and finally body movements.[8] Often, you can tell how someone is feeling based on their body movements alone. If you wear your emotions on your sleeve, then this is definitely a property you want to invest in. If you are not sharing your feelings, something may be preventing you from enjoying your life, and it might come out in your body language and reactions. The hope is that you can get to the point where you are happy with how you feel and think, and can therefore hold your head up high and say bring it on!

Keep in mind that if you make any attempt to cut any of these corners there is the chance you will go to "the Consequence Center" to strategize again and rethink your game plan. Additionally, there is the "communication to others," the utility square. Therefore, you may land on the square and the card says "You sent an e-mail with all your thoughts to the wrong person. Go back to social balance and mend that relationship." Another example could be "You have engaged in three straight months of healthy sharing and reflecting your feelings with a friend. Proceed to the Happy Birthday square and collect more time," (better known as two hundred dollars).

Then you proceed to roll the dice again and you make that final lap around the fourth row of properties. Where you are now in your life will depend on who you are, but in this example it is physical balance.[9]

For many people this is one of the hardest, most

challenging areas. Physical balance can be divided into two sections: eating habits and exercise. Eating habits are the two most expensive properties on the board. It is often difficult for people to balance all aspects of life and maintain healthy eating habits. It is too easy to slip or be unaware that what you are eating is actually doing more harm than good. As great as exercise is, if you are not eating properly you are working against everything you exercise for.

Within eating habits there are two properties: understanding your own body's needs, and the implementation of a healthy and consistent eating plan. It is important to realize that there are different body types and your body's needs will be different from those of others. To establish and maintain a regular and healthy eating routine, it might be helpful to keep a record of what you eat and when. Sure, you can treat yourself every so often, but making sure you maintain a proper eating schedule is essential. Many people struggle with good eating habits for various reasons (e.g., lack of motivation, cost, time, etc.), but healthy eating is a possibility.

Do not forget activities, goal-setting[4], regular exercise[9], and stretching. These activities may include scholastic sports, adult clubs, or some form of daily exercise. It is most important to make these activities a regular part of your day at least three to four days of the week.[9] Lastly, always changing the exercise plan can be crucial for optimal success. If you do the same thing every week for fifty-two weeks, you use the same areas of the body, neglect others, and you may become bored with the routine or injured. Changing your regimen will help you keep exercising. Therefore, you are to have ownership of the property that allows you to change your exercise plan. Maybe in the winter you play ice hockey and in the summer you golf, play baseball, or run.

Whatever the case, be sure to exercise regularly, monitor your goal attainment, and always change the routine to ensure you are one step ahead of your game. Because as we all know, the square in between the two most expensive properties is a penalty square. Therefore, this exercise and balance stuff does not come easy, so be prepared to pay the price.

There you have it: the reasoning behind why and how to make every attempt to monopolize your life in all four aspects of balance. It is crucial to understand the analogy before delving further into this book, so that you can design your own board game for your life and decide how to allocate the four rows. Which row would be first, which would be last, and what falls in between? To win the game, it may help to balance each and every aspect throughout life. The metaphor of the board game will resurface throughout the book, so feel free to return to it throughout and personalize it each time.

Life is a game of chance, of preparation, and of learning how to properly respond to the obstacles you will face. Life delivers setbacks, but if you are ready, you will have a great chance of overcoming them. The ability to remain sturdy on our feet throughout the setbacks and joys is based on the recognition that it is not your legs that are holding you back. It is a proper balance of the physical, the emotional, the social, and the professional aspects of your life and the choices you make throughout that will make the difference. Together, these will be referred to as the four pillars of balance.

Be aware that success is a personal and all-encompassing definition that takes into account family, work life, and your personal choices. In the following chapters, each of the pillars that contributes to balancing life will be outlined, along with how it can effectively be approached and personalized.

Notes Page
Thoughts? Feelings? Intentions? Actions?

_____

_____

_____

_____

_____

_____

_____

_____

_____

_____

_____

_____

_____

_____

_____

_____

_____

_____

_____

_____

_____

_____

CHAPTER 2
Putting Your Mental Skills to the Test

"Just as your car runs more smoothly and requires less energy to go faster and farther when the wheels are in perfect alignment, you perform better when your thoughts, feelings, emotions, goals, and values are in balance."
~Brian Tracy

t *is* possible, you *can* achieve it: you *can* be successful at work, at home, and in your relationships while remaining physically fit. There are a variety of effective techniques that can be used to make the above not just a concept, but a reality. It is important to transfer the same motivating techniques you use at work or school to everyday life to help create balance. The aim is to use a variety of mental skills that will help you balance the four main pillars of your life: physical, mental or emotional, social, and academic or professional. These mental skills involve self-talk[1], relaxation[2], imagery[3], goal-setting[4], paying attention[10] to what may increase worry in specific situations and in life, and communication[5] (which will be discussed in later chapters). The main purpose of consistently adding psychological tools into your life is to increase your motivation and ability to succeed. The chapter will outline these tools to help paint the picture for you and how you can use these skills every day.

Self-talk

Self-talk[1] is a mental activity that involves having a positive belief in your potential. It can also act as encouragement. The purpose is to help you manage your own negative thoughts and translate them into more positive ones by communicating with yourself. If you can tell yourself there is potential, you will then seek to attain that potential. Negative self-talk[1], on the other hand, inhibits you when it becomes constant self-criticism. Self-talk can have the power to influence choices, actions, and self-esteem. It is first important to be aware of negative self-talk.

Start keeping track of instances of negative self-talk. Write them down each time you catch yourself. Some examples of negative self-talk are: "It's a stupid game anyway," "It doesn't really matter," "I don't think I should attempt this because I won't succeed like my friends always do," "I don't have the same skills as the other people to do this, I'll just end up looking ridiculous," "If I add a comment to this meeting, what if others don't agree, or worse what if they all laugh at me?", "I'll never get it, maybe I should just not even bother," "Everybody else is doing better than me anyway."

How you talk to yourself before and during a test or any potential perceived intimidating interaction may influence your performance. It is essential to engage in positive self-talk[1] as you process your thoughts. Doing so may help you process thoughts in a rational step-wise method in which you can translate your own internalized thinking into action. When you start to hear yourself using negative self-talk, ask yourself "What proof do I have that I am not going to succeed, or that I am not as good as the other people?"

By using a more positive frame of mind, your negative thoughts can be converted into affirmations. Some examples (and there are many) include: "This test is important to me and my progress in school. I can do it if I breathe and take one step at a time," "It's okay to be nervous, and it's okay to mess up on one question. I just need to take a deep breath and try the next question without getting hysterical," "I'm just going to do the best I can," "Hey, I'm doing okay here on this test. I'm definitely a little nervous, but I believe I have this thing under control," "It's okay if my classmates finish before me and work faster than me. I am going to continue to work at my own speed until I am finished," "I can get through this test without falling apart, I feel proud," "It's okay if I encounter opposition; perhaps I'll open their eyes to another view, or maybe they'll teach me something I didn't consider."[1]

When you are in a situation where you doubt yourself, write down your negative self-talk and your unhelpful thoughts and rewrite them as positive statements and thoughts. Merely considering the positive perspective, you may alter your actions for the better. Even writing down your thought or taking a moment to consider why you doubt your ability will allow you to see it does not truly have any merit; nor does it represent what the likely result will be. If you were the spectator watching someone else in your shoes, would you react the way the people watching you would react? Your thoughts and how you communicate them to yourself influence how you will act. Focus on what is really happening and what you are really capable of, versus what you think is happening.

Attentional Control

Attentional control[10] involves your ability to focus on specific tasks without being distracted. When you lose interest in various things you will begin to mentally drift, also known as day-dreaming. As a consequence, this distraction can disrupt your learning and interaction with others around you. One technique to increase your ability to remain focused is the use of positive reinforcement.[11] Positive reinforcement involves being rewarded for engaging in a desired behavior in the hope that it will be repeated.[11] Engaging in effective attentional control may help to improve your ability to complete certain tasks and reduce distracting behaviors.

Another technique that helps reduce distractions and increase attentional focus is the use of relaxation[2], both in the home and at school or the office. Too often you will come into your office, send e-mails, check the web, search your favorite sites, and before you know it two hours have gone by and you have not accomplished a thing. However, engaging in regular relaxation techniques upon or prior to entering the office may help you calm down and stay focused, and can lead to greater productivity.[2] Staying focused in class may help you retain more of the material presented. Focusing on conversations will benefit your interactions. And when you give your full attention to conversations with other people, you will notice that stronger connections develop.

Relaxation

By engaging in simple methods of relaxation you will be able to settle the mind, body, and spirit.[2] The settled mind may provide you with the realization that you actually have the motivation and ability to succeed. Relaxation is an activity and a state of mind and body connection that is intended to decrease your tension and anxiety.[2] The idea is to acknowledge and then diminish stress. Furthermore, it can increase an individual's positive behavior and, in turn, increase chances of success. Thus, this tool has a positive effect on all four pillars of balance.

Some forms of relaxation include initial work by Edmond Jacobson and his technique of progressive muscle relaxation (PMR).[2] PMR involves going through each part of your body and internally squeezing the specific body part (similar to 'making a muscle'), holding the tension for approximately five to seven seconds (e.g., one Mississippi, two Mississippi, etc.), and then releasing it for twenty to thirty seconds. While releasing the tension, you are to feel your muscles become more relaxed. The hope is that you will do each part twice before moving to the next body part. Starting with the face and moving down to the toes, according to Jacobson's theory, you can relax anywhere from five to sixteen body parts (see *Appendix A* for an example). Another option is to start at your toes and slowly focus on each muscle until you reach your eyes and then your forehead. Complete the exercise with a nice long stretch and a deep breath.

The idea is that you verbally express what has been accomplished, what needs more work, and receive optimal rest opportunities. Engaging in relaxation can prevent disruptions in class or the office, and promote a more stress-free individual.[2] You can feel better about who you are, what you have accomplished, and what you have the ability to accomplish. The concept of *nap-time* ended once you left kindergarten, but relaxation techniques are a practical alternative that can last a lifetime.

Take ten minutes out of each day to close your eyes, drain your concerns, your tasks at hand, any negative thoughts, any topics of stress, and any frustration. Mentally going through the body and determining what part of the body feels most stressed, tense, or irritated can help you clear those feelings. Starting with your head and moving to your feet, spending a certain amount of time on each muscle group and limb in your body, may help you to better identify the location of the most stress. The relaxation minutes should be spent focusing on each muscle in your body. Just ten minutes out of your day can make you calmer and more grounded in your environment. If you have time for more than ten minutes, then by all means take that time.

Imagery

In conjunction with relaxation, another important skill is guided imagery.[3] Imagery uses both mental pictures and relaxation to enhance one's physical well-being and mood.[3] Imagery is visualizing a scene or a situation in which a task will be completed. Once in a relaxed state, the idea is to imagine how certain academic and/or professional or even social situations may be approached. This creates a feeling of readiness and control of situations you may encounter.

Imagery can create a form of mental connection between the mind and body.[3] Engaging in imagery may contribute to a more relaxed state, decreased stress, lower blood pressure, and may help contribute to a stronger immune system.[3] By imagining how you will accomplish certain tasks, you can control worry and concentrate on the task at hand.

There are a number of different types of imagery and it is essential to understand each of them to ensure you are using it to your best advantage. Pain control imagery involves a technique in which you concentrate on a specific area of physical pain and by focusing upon it, slowly decrease it.[3] Relaxation imagery is a variation of what Johannes Schultz and Wolfgang Luthe referred to as autogenic training.[3] The process involves imagining a safe and relaxed place and slowly allowing your mind to place yourself in the warmth of that setting.[3]

Regardless of the type of imagery you choose, the main thing is guiding your thoughts and your mind to that state of relaxation. Effective use of imagery will dampen any surprises you may be faced with and will enable you to see how obstacles may be confronted. Therefore, simply mentally acting out the scenario, you will be more prepared and motivated to engage in the situation. When you imagine how a setting will look, it will not seem so unfamiliar when the time comes to perform.

Goal-setting

Goal-setting[4] increases your realization of what you most desire, need, and want, on both the professional or academic and non-professional or non-academic levels. Realizing goals provides an opportunity to plan for them and increases the chances that you will accomplish them. Make sure you can measure your progress and attain your goals within a desirable time-frame. If your progress is not measurable and a time-frame cannot be applied, then it may be a dream, as opposed to a goal. The last thing you want to do is set unrealistic goals that will be difficult to reach.

Write your goals down, and ask yourself why you want to set such goals. Prepare for obstacles that may interfere with successful attainment, change them accordingly, ensure you have some form of a support network as you progress, and make sure you work for the goals you set. To balance everything that life throws your way, learning how to effectively set goals so you know where you are, where you want to go, and how far you have come can have a greater impact on your life than you may realize.

Referring back to the board game, these are properties to your life that you do not need to have ownership over, but as you may be able to see, it can definitely help. The above psychological tools may enhance your relative success rate. It is important to outline what you want to accomplish and begin planning how you will accomplish it. Furthermore, it is essential to always be altering your desires and beliefs to maintain health and balance. If you focus too much on one goal and the desired outcome is not attained, your motivation may suffer.

It is imperative that you are honest with yourself, and that you remain patient, focused, and aware of your own abilities, as well as of which, if any, of the psychological skills are important for you to embrace. Above all, remember that being realistic is important, and you must consider all of the circumstances independently involved in each situation. If you stay motivated, focused, relaxed, and set small attainable goals, you have a much greater chance at achieving *your* optimal balanced success.

Quick Points

- Self-talk – tell yourself you are capable, worthy, and will succeed; and if you do not, that is okay; it is not the end of the world. Talk to yourself in ways that will be helpful.
- Attentional control – actively pay attention to what you are doing and focus on one task at a time. Know that you will eventually get to the other tasks, but for now, one task at a time.
- Relaxation – take a step back before engaging in a stressful event, breathe, and pay attention to where your body is most tense. Do not ignore the pressure.
- Imagery – imagine what the stressful event might look like without excessively worrying about it. Imagine the sights, sounds, and smells of the area. Prepare yourself for how you might react, and realize thoughts are just thoughts.
- Goal-setting – set small goals that you can attain and praise yourself every time you do so. Understand that you may not achieve all of your goals, but that does not mean you cannot achieve others. Be sure to set both process and outcome goals and adjust them when necessary.

Notes Page
Thoughts? Feelings? Intentions? Actions?

_____

_____

_____

_____

_____

_____

_____

_____

_____

_____

_____

_____

_____

_____

_____

_____

_____

_____

_____

_____

_____

_____

_____

CHAPTER 3
Physical Balance –
With More Than Just
Two Feet on the Ground

"You will miss 100% of the shots you don't take."
~Wayne Gretzky

Professional athlete and Canadian legend Wayne Gretzky was often asked how was he able to practice ice hockey seven hours every day as a child. He pointed out that he did not see it as a task. He spent so long on the ice because he saw it as an enjoyable way to use his time. For me, athletic pursuits were much the same.

While going through elementary school, I was enrolled in swimming year round, ice hockey in the winter, and either soccer or baseball in the summer. A quick message to kids and parents: The key to finding a physical balance in your life during elementary and high school is to try everything you can and then pick the few that you enjoy the most.

The tendency is for kids to drop out or change activities halfway through as they begin to realize what they enjoy most. Thus, the key is to focus on getting involved with as many different sports or activities as you can. Interests will likely blossom in at least one sport or activity if you allow for it. As with many aspects of your life, you need to see what you do not want before you know for certain what you do want. The notion of a physically balanced life begins with the desire and choice to enroll in athletics. Engaging in some form of regular physical fitness can do wonders for your physical growth, confidence, and cardiovascular health.[9]

When you are younger your bones need to grow and become healthier and stronger. Physical activity in early life may contribute to enhanced health later in life, too. Involving yourself in various physical activities early in life can train your body to withstand more intensity. I look at my grandfather, who was an athlete in college, sustained injuries when he became older, and recovered from those injuries much faster because of his body's ability to respond. Therefore, if you choose to continue with athletics, your body will be able to accept the rigorous workload later in life. If the intensity of some sports is intimidating for you, look into less intense activities or engage in the challenge. As long as there is some form of physical activity, your body is getting the attention it deserves.

It is often tempting to put off exercise because you feel too tired or because you believe that you do not have time or money to join health clubs or team sports. However, it is important to find the time and motivation for an exercise program. Additionally, include exercises that may not require as much money to participate in (e.g., running or walking). Turning off the television to go out and exercise is often a good place to start.

Remember, the barriers to exercise are a choice. Regardless of your ability, there is always some form of exercise you can engage in. It is a matter of making the choice at any given time and telling yourself *I can*. Be creative and go outside and play.

Staying in shape does not require one to be in top physical condition and have an ideal body type. A 300-pound football player may be in similar shape as a 130-pound swimmer. They are simply different body types. Their heart rate, blood flow, and breathing rate may all be normal. Therefore, when they run up five flights of stairs they are not out of breath. People rely on elevators and escalators to do the work for them and consequently get used to not having to use their muscles to move. There is an easy way to avoid being too tired, finding time, and all the while not paying a dime.

Regular exercise does not require much; it is the motivation that requires most of the energy.[9] Every day when you get home from school or work, you can take forty-five minutes to engage in some form of physical activity or regular exercise. If you are signed up for Little League sports, then chances are you already engage in three days of physical fitness. If Little League sports are not your cup of tea, or you are beyond that age group, then try working within your environment. Try running up and down stairs inside or outside for twenty minutes, followed by push-ups, and then back to the stairs for ten more minutes. The routine can be completed with a two- or three-minute cool-down to have your heart rate return back to normal, and at least five to ten minutes of proper stretching before and after. If you need the motivation to do such activity, then play your top ten songs on your iPod, or whatever hand-held music machine you have access to, and that in and of itself will get you excited.[12] By the time the ten songs are over, you will have completed your exercise! Remember to slowly increase your effort and duration of the activity in moderation.

Therefore, if you start with twenty minutes, every two weeks move up an additional three minutes. Adding the extra one hundred and eighty seconds will make a huge difference in your progress. If you are beyond the age of Little League sports, there are adult leagues. If you need to work on your own schedule, sign up for the gym. Keep in mind that signing up does not generate exercise; you do actually have to go to the facility. Thus, look into classes they offer, and if you prefer to work out independently, you can still set your own goals. However, do make note that having a friend or significant other who exercises with you can help maintain the motivation. To help optimize the physical portion of your balance, a healthy combination of weight training and cardiovascular exercise can give you the energy to focus on other facets of your life. For a sample exercise plan, see *Appendix B*.

To see slight, but significant progress, do not forget to set small goals that are within reach.[4] Take advantage of every opportunity to increase your stamina. If you are at the mall, use the stairs to get to the next floor. If you need to get something from the store that is a quick drive or a ten-minute walk, choose the walk. Unfortunately, we have become a society reliant on efficiency and convenience. We take every opportunity to make things easier in less time. Put in the effort; you will thank yourself for it later.

For example, internet shopping eliminates any steps we would take to the mall or local store. Walking, instead of driving, sounds simple. However, as a society, the only movement that seems to be happening is moving further away from effort and closer to someone or some technology taking care of it for us. Maximize every opportunity you have to engage in physical activity, and you will meet your mark or desired goal for each week, by taking more steps. Instead of trying to find the closest spot to the door, park the farthest away so you have to walk to the door. When you get in the store, take the stairs instead of the escalators or elevators. It is likely that the more time you take to exercise now, the less time you will spend in the hospital waiting room attending to potential health concerns.

What contributes to a sluggish attitude? Two simple words: fast food. It is cheap and tastes great. There is so much salt and sugar in every item you eat at any fast food restaurant that it keeps you coming back for more. Two more words to pay attention to: portion size. It is shocking how little attention people pay to the effects of fast food and the amount they are eating. I am not saying eliminate it from your life, but just make different choices while you are there. If you are a parent and going to a fast food restaurant is the easiest thing to do every now and then, limit what your children can order and how often you take this easy route. You are the parent, they are not.

Make an effort to eat at home and provide healthier options with many colors on the plate. Of course, children like snacks, need sugar, and will eat anything that is covered in chocolate. However, if those options are not available to them at home, they may be more inclined to eat what is available. Instead of offering or eating food that is loaded with calories and grease, you may have to diminish the delicious to increase the nutritious. Eating at a fast food restaurant or using the drive-thru more often than you exercise may be a sign to change the behavior to help create physical balance in your life. If you can choose healthier options, you will maintain your physical goals as time progresses.

Now that you have made a choice to eat healthier, what do you eat and how often? The key is to eat smaller meals more often.[13] We all seem to be so busy throughout the day, leading us to grab whatever is quick, easy, cheap, and tastes good. However, the effects on your body of eating the cheapest greasiest food can be disastrous.[13] Your body's digestion is usually fastest throughout the bulk of your day, from approximately eight o'clock in the morning until four o'clock in the afternoon. Thus, by eating after nine o'clock in the evening, you might not be able to fall asleep as quickly because your body is still digesting. Because your metabolism is slower, eating late in the day may contribute to weight gain. Therefore, it is important to consider not just what you eat, but also when you eat.

A standard schedule for the *average* North American lifestyle is provided in the following section, and also see *Appendix C* for a more detailed eating plan. The appendix outlines a simple suggestion for healthier eating habits en route to creating a balanced physical self. The ideal is for you to eat immediately after you wake up (and no, not just coffee), then a small mid-morning snack, a hearty lunch, a mid-afternoon snack, a colorful dinner, and a later snack. Note that the time slots for when you eat are mere approximations and can be adjusted according to various schedules. As long as the eating starts first thing in the morning and finishes a few hours before you go to bed, you are doing wonders.

Begin with breakfast (e.g., cereal, eggs, or oatmeal with serving sizes of fiber) at seven or eight o'clock in the morning. Follow it up with a snack at ten-thirty (e.g., granola bar, fruit, vegetable, etc.). At lunch, replace fried food with an alternative, such as fruit, vegetables, and a sandwich. You do not need to eliminate fried foods entirely. Remember, the body does need certain oils. The key is for you to be aware of what you are eating. Instead of pop, choose a bottle of water. The positive effects of water, in addition to eliminating the sugar rush and inevitable crash of pop, makes it a practical alternative.

As you attempt to balance your eating, be sure not to overeat. Many times people will overeat at lunch because they did not have breakfast or the mid-morning snack. Sometimes people overeat just because food is there (e.g., holidays, weddings, or bar mitzvahs).

Unfortunately, as many have experienced, overeating can result in feeling sluggish and tired throughout the latter portion of the day. The resulting lethargic feelings may lead to less productivity (see Thanksgiving and many festive holiday meals for prime examples).

Therefore, eat a smaller lunch (but not too small, where you end up famished before the afternoon snack or dinner), minimize what is fried, and substitute your beverage with water. Have water and a snack around three or four in the afternoon. Make every attempt to choose a healthier snack, and remember those five-dollar energy bars that have plenty of protein also have plenty of sugar! By the time six o'clock comes around, your body will be ready for its next meal.

Dinner is the meal that seems to be the *nail in the coffin* for people who usually overeat, in large part because they have not eaten all day. First of all, make every attempt to eat dinner before eight o'clock in the evening. Second, do your best to include some bread, vegetables, meat or tofu, some form of dairy, and above all, fiber. If you are restricted from eating meat with milk, then have the milk dinners on a separate day from the meat dinners. Throughout the meal, try to have two or three cups of water. Again, for a more detailed meal plan see *Appendix C* and adjust accordingly if allergies interfere with the suggested items (e.g., nuts, gluten intolerance).

The tendency is for those out of grade school to go to bed after eleven o'clock in the evening and those in grade school before eleven o'clock. Therefore, plan your meal accordingly and try and eat the last meal at least three hours before you head to bed. If for whatever reason you are up late or coming home late from an extracurricular activity, then feel free to eat a light, simple meal — say cereal, fruit, or yogurt. You will fall asleep without hunger pangs but will not have the food weighing you down.

Lastly, be aware of your portion sizes. I have noticed that often restaurants will actually be serving you double or even triple the portion size you would be eating at home. Furthermore, they load the recipe with extra oils and salts to add to the taste. Therefore, be certain you know your limits: just because you ordered it, that does not mean you have to eat it all. Decide beforehand to take some of it home and have it for lunch the next day. Stepping back for a moment during your meal or putting your fork down between bites every so often may be a way to help prevent you from feeling the regret of overeating. If overeating is a concern for you, pay close attention to the size of the plate you are using, as changing it may help, and ask yourself why you are choosing to overeat.

Prevention will result in retention of your physical self. The more prevention you take by engaging in daily physical fitness and eating smaller, well-balanced meals more often throughout your day, the more you may retain your energy. My friend Dave once said, "Change is not always easy, but necessary nevertheless." Even though it is difficult, you have the choice to change your lifestyle now, before your doctor tells you that one more order of fries and your ticker will stop ticking, or your dentist tells you one more candy bar and it will be dentures at twenty. If your significant other or close friends are choosing to not eat healthy or exercise regularly, that does not mean you have to follow their lead. You make your choices, and they can make theirs. Say it to yourself: This my life... and I will make my choices.

Referring back to the game board with physical balance being the most difficult to attain, it is important that you realize the information above is available to anyone; you just have to tailor the elements to the resources that you have. Therefore, pay close attention to how much you want to *invest* in regular exercise and well-planned healthy eating en route to balancing the physical properties in your life.

Quick Points

- Regular physical activity at least three days per week and realize that barriers to exercise are there because of how you perceive them; you can get through them.
- Eat five small well-balanced meals each day.
- Set small goals that realistically can be achieved.
- Reward yourself every ten days.
- Choose healthier options at fast food restaurants.
- Be aware of the portion sizes.
- Do not compare yourself to others. Everyone is built differently, so each person adhering to the suggestions above may have to tweak it one way or another.

Notes Page
Thoughts? Feelings? Intentions? Actions?

_____

_____

_____

_____

_____

_____

_____

_____

_____

_____

_____

_____

_____

_____

_____

_____

_____

_____

_____

_____

_____

CHAPTER 4
Emotional and Mental Balance – Working With the Inside for the Best Outside

"People are disturbed not by things, but by the views they take on them."
~Epictetus, *The Enchiridion*

Life has a tendency to create barriers along our paths. It is important we deal with these obstacles and try to overcome them. However, much of our success in how we do overcome these barriers emerges from how we *choose* to view the situation. To optimistically and proactively approach our challenges, it is important that we view how they will ultimately benefit us. Hurt and pain can be seen as an opportunity for challenge or development, rather than as defeat. Therefore, barriers in your life are a prime opportunity to put your true character to the test. You are ultimately left with a *choice* regarding how to respond to the difficult situation.

That which contributes to you feeling good on the inside has the tendency to direct how you feel on the outside. If something in life is bringing you down, (e.g., a failed math test, a broken heart, or being rejected by a job or a school), it becomes quite difficult to separate the inside thoughts and feelings from the outside reactions and how others see your sadness and pain. Having the ability to make a distinction and make yourself aware of what you are truly feeling is not an easy task.

Many people have the tendency to displace their feelings. For example, you may be discouraged, frustrated, and disappointed because you were not hired for a certain job. You might react negatively to any little thing. You might take out your disappointment on a friend, a parent, a sibling, or a stranger on the street. You are projecting your inner emotions upon someone else. We all endure negative feelings, situations, and life-changing events that often present our biggest growing opportunities.

Sure, certain thoughts, like "I will never feel such love and passion again!" or "Why did this have to happen to me?" may come to you. When you engage in any task or relationship, you hope to put everything into it: love, devotion, attention, challenge, and affection. However, when something to which you have devoted considerable time and attention does not end as you had hoped, you begin to question how you can ever get past such a negative event or feeling.

You can if you *choose* to. It is important not to ignore negative experiences. Experiencing the negative is as important as embracing the positive. After all, both are moments of time from which you can learn.

Many have used the cliché that the grass is always greener on the other side, especially when we are experiencing a negative life event. How do you think the grass becomes greener? Let it rain; it is okay. Feel the rain run through your hands, head, and heart. When a negative experience happens, it is essential to pay close attention to it, making yourself aware of what your thoughts and feelings are about it.[14] It is important that you take time to look deep inside yourself and ask: What do I need to do and want to do to optimize myself as a person? It is not an easy process to truly experience hurt.

You are allowing yourself to look for things to change to be the "best me." Of course not all moments are going to be easy. You may experience a bundle of feelings like nausea, loss of appetite, loneliness, fear, regret, and confusion. You might also do some absurd things that are unlike you, but that is just part of the process of experiencing the emotions in their truest form. The reality is that during a time of hurt, you are not yourself, and that is okay as long as you are attempting to explore why. Do not be afraid to experience the feeling, because it will pass with time. After all, time never really stops.

You may feel so helpless at times that you have no idea what to do. These thoughts and events are in the bigger picture. They are moments that will pass and in due time become less frequent as you heal and reemerge as yourself again. Unfortunately, experiences like these cannot be avoided or hurried by swiping your credit card through a magical machine. They happen and it is important that you choose not to avoid them or cover them up (e.g., burying yourself in work or starting a new relationship too quickly).

Choose to begin the new day on your feet. Remember that you do not need to live for tomorrow or for yesterday. Today is your day. That is not saying live like today is your last, as that can instill fear, panic, regret, worry, and the like. However, it is saying that you should try as hard as you can to truly be present in your moments, both the good and the bad. Live for today and take time to experience all that comes with the now, including your thoughts. What has happened has already taken place; what might happen is unknown. What you do know is the now. Focus on experiencing it, because anything can change in a moment. It may be one negative event, but that does not determine who you are as a whole person – it is just one single part of you. Too often when a negative event happens we focus so much on it that we tend to ignore all the other positive events in our lives.

Understand that whatever happens, you are learning more about yourself and how you respond to difficulty in your life. The time you take to understand your reactions to difficulties will help you understand who you are, and will help you approach future experiences with more perspective. The more you choose to look deep inside your thoughts and emotions, the more you will be aware of what triggers them.

Thus, while negative incidents may hurt, and may

create a sense of helplessness, pay close attention to how you respond, and realize that one isolated incident does not define you. You do not want negative feelings and thoughts of one event to control your whole day. In times of painful experiences, keep expressing the thoughts as they emerge. Doing this will help you bring your reality to life and realize not just where you have been, but who you want to be after you emerge from the experience.

Sure, you will engage in random activities, go on vacations, or bury your head in your work to distract yourself, which can be important. However, it is equally important to be mindful[14] of how you are feeling, and thus check in with yourself constantly. By becoming aware that creating more work for yourself or running from a situation does not remove the situation can do wonders. This avoidance tactic is a method of escape, and may only help in the short-term.

Everyone has the ability to recover from life's setbacks at a different pace. Go at the speed that feels appropriate, take the turns you want, and try to enjoy the ride. In time, you will be able to smile, laugh, dance, and breathe. Talk to a trusted friend, family member, teacher, therapist, colleague, or coach about your emotions and feelings. Vent. Do not hold back. If you are not feeling like yourself, pay attention to that and ask yourself why. Do not be afraid to confront the negative feelings you are having or that have resurfaced from years past. Check in with yourself, but above all take ownership of the feeling, and know you will recover if you allow yourself to think about it and feel it.

How do you become aware of your emotions to

help give you a better state of mind? They may be expressed in at least three different ways: verbally[15], physically,[16] or in writing.[17] If you are the type of person who has no problem saying anything, you are usually the person at the party who does not have any discretion and says what is on your mind at both the right time and wrong time, then obviously expressing yourself verbally is not the issue. However, if you are speaking a lot about surface-related issues to avoid deeper emotions, then it is essential to pay close attention to that as well.

Verbal

If you choose to ignore negative thoughts and emotions that have been with you for days, months, or years, you may be living your past, missing your present, and may never truly be able to embrace your future. Express yourself verbally to someone you can trust and respect, and with whom you feel comfortable. What you are attempting to do is understand where the root of the emotional distraction is coming from. You can attain this by hearing yourself express this out loud. You are not trying to blame anyone; you are trying to locate the root of why you are so emotionally bothered, as it may not be directly due to an incident, but something beyond that has been ignored for years. It is essential to make an attempt to pinpoint the exact reason for the unhappiness. Usually it is not the obvious issues that cause the distress. Be honest, go deeper, and think harder about the real reason why you are distressed and how one incident may just bring out the major issue, perhaps from your past.

It is okay to be honest with yourself as to how you are truly feeling and thinking, and communicate that effectively. Many say and believe they are honest, but yet when they verbalize their thoughts, true honesty does not emerge because of the fear of possibly hurting someone. The hardest part about honest communication is saying what your mind might already know that your heart has not been informed of yet, or vice versa. Feel free to let your heart and mind engage in a conversation; the hope is they can get along. See what you can do about telling someone how you feel; then work on how you can change the negative feeling and prevent it from happening again in the future. Detailed methods of verbal expression to alleviate emotional stress will be explained later in the chapter.

Physical

The second major form of creating awareness of emotional distress is a physical reaction.[16] If, for whatever reason, you are not so comfortable with expressing yourself verbally, then a physical response is a possibility, but not by bullying.[16] For many cultures, verbalizing your thoughts, feelings, and emotions is taboo.[15] However, there is always the alternative of physical expression. Be aware that physical expression is not physical violence. Physical expression can be experienced through regular exercise.[9]

An issue causing you emotional distress can be

released through physical exertion while engaging in some form of self-talk[1] to help uncover what is really bothering you. As defined earlier, self-talk[1] is a form of communication within the self that coaches the individual on the spot. For example, when a tennis player is looking to serve an ace into the opposing court, he or she may say to themselves: "Okay, come on now — right down the line, here we go, just make this shot and we'll win the set."

If releasing some form of emotion with physical exertion is most effective for you, then combine that exertion with self-talk[1] to create inner awareness. An excellent example of this is running.[9] As you are running around a track, around your block, or on the treadmill, talk to yourself and open up what is most troublesome. You may find that as you begin to talk about what bothers you, your intensity level will increase. You may start to run faster as your heart rate increases. Therefore, whatever begins to trigger the most emotion and adrenaline in the moment is the most likely cause of the emotional distress. You will find that after long enough periods of engaged self-talk, the crux of the issue will emerge.

For example, when you are at the dentist and the drill touches the most sensitive part of your tooth, something inside of you responds quickly with a jolt. It is the same type of scenario with internal thoughts and feelings. When you engage in self-talk and exploration of the emotion, at one point or another you will hit that emotional nerve comparable to that at the dentist. As soon as that emotional nerve is touched you have to stop, step back for a moment, and say to yourself: "This is it, this is what has been causing a lot of my stress."

What tends to happen is that the stress is attributed to a variety of causes. The reason for the distress, however, can be hidden or avoided only for so long. Eventually with enough self-talk[1] while physically engaging in an activity, the truth behind the emotion may be revealed. Another technique is to look at yourself in the mirror when thinking about your emotions. Watch your reactions when you speak of a certain person, worry, or situation. Pay close attention to how you are reacting to everything you are thinking about. Taking the time to think about your thoughts and how they are directing your feelings can help you to better understand why and when certain emotions present themselves. If you are feeling down or upset about a bothersome issue, the key to becoming aware of the root of the real problem is not to release some form of physical abuse on someone or something. That does not resolve the issue; nor does it let you rationally understand it.

The water pouring into a strainer might temporarily fill the strainer, but eventually it runs out again and you are back where you started. The same applies to a physical response to an emotional issue. For example, you hit someone or something because you are angry. That might provide you some release temporarily, but eventually the issue creeps up again because you have not truly confronted or made yourself aware of it. It is essential to know the significant difference between physical exertion (e.g., releasing emotion while engaging in a physical activity) and physical abuse (e.g., engaging in a physical reaction in response to an underlying issue or immediate incident).

Written

Written expression is another excellent form of awareness; it is the expression of one's most intimate and inner feelings.[17] People tend not to express how they are truly feeling because of the fear of hearing themselves say something they do not want to hear, or because they do not know how to verbalize what they are feeling. Therefore, write your feelings down on paper, type them in a document, or even type them in an e-mail you send to yourself. Written communication allows you to express how you are feeling[5] and gives you the freedom to retract your statements by deleting, altering, or crossing out. The attractiveness of written expression is that it allows you to be creative.

Furthermore, written communication allows you to commit to statements and thoughts, go back to these statements, and reread what you wrote and what you were feeling at that time in your life. If you write out your thoughts and use them to set small attainable goals for yourself, you can monitor your progress via written communication. It is one thing to write your own thoughts, feelings, and emotions on paper or type them and keep them private. It is another thing to share what you have written or typed. If you share, be sure you do so only with a trusted friend who will respect your privacy and will understand and appreciate your expression.

Sometimes we want to write e-mails telling someone everything we think, when in fact they do not care to read it all, and they will reply with "sounds good." If you do plan to share your feelings through written word, know your audience. Sometimes it may be best to write or type out all of your thoughts and then, depending on your audience, summarize if need be. I am saying this only because I have heard too many folks tell me: "I wrote out everything I was thinking and she or he said nothing in response." To prevent disappointment, write out the thoughts for and with you. If you choose to share those thoughts, be aware of whom you choose to send them to.

Be careful of when you do type out your thoughts and feelings in an e-mail, being aware of the ramifications of sending messages over some form of wireless network that may not be entirely private. The recipient may not be the only reader! The same holds true for social networking sites, which are a common method of communication. Many people will post pictures, stories, and thoughts on those web pages. Be careful with respect to what you publicize, as once it is on the internet, anyone can access it a lot easier than you may ever realize.

Your life and emotions are your business; be careful as to whom you trust with the information you are sharing, as it is your business. When it comes to your feelings and emotions, be careful of what you send, and to whom. Expressing your emotions — verbally[15], physically[16], or in writing[17] – may help to alleviate additional stressors and decrease the amount of unwanted mental baggage you may unwillingly be carrying around with you. Understanding the positive thoughts that you need and the negative thoughts you do not need may help distinguish between mental baggage and mental luggage.

Distinguishing Between Luggage and Baggage

It is important to better understand what makes these two terms different. Luggage includes all the items you *need* to bring with you to carry out your daily mental and emotional functioning. Baggage, on the other hand, includes those items that you obsess over. They tend to distress you and those around you. These items are those that you *choose* to bring with you. These items include many aspects of life that seem out of your hands, that you cannot control, and those that are creating dysfunction and disturbance that you may be ignoring.

To better understand the distinction between luggage and baggage, pay attention both to how you travel and how others travel when boarding an airplane. Please note that these protocols may change as airlines charge more for the number of bags one is allowed to bring onboard. Those who pack what they *need* will have it all fit into one average-sized suitcase. They know exactly what items they will need during their time away. Conversely, those who bring an excess have not thought through what is most necessary, and often *choose* to bring everything. Knowing someone has baggage cautions your approach, as that person may be carrying troubling issues or experiences. Regardless of whether it is baggage or luggage, the bottom line is it is the *choice* in how you perceive what is most important to bring with you on your journey throughout life.

The key behind feelings and emotions that can help connect much of your distress is how you choose to think about the distressing events. It all begins with how and what you choose to tell yourself. As mentioned previously, the use of verbal communication is imperative to understanding your distress.[15] Thus, begin with telling yourself that regardless of any distress that is occurring or will occur, above all you like yourself, and you are a valuable individual. Yes, distress happens and negative experiences will occur, but above all you are still okay. If it helps, include random short motivating phrases as text messages to yourself to read when you need reminders.

Furthermore, communicate to yourself that it is okay to take risks, even if that means you might fail. Failure is only a part of the process that will help direct you down the right road. Talk to yourself. If you are not feeling like you usually do, ask yourself why. Ask yourself what thoughts are creating the distress, and what methods you can use to overcome the distress. Above all, ask yourself if the thought you are having right now is helpful, and if it is not — change it!

An effective five-step method of thinking about your thoughts was originally proposed in the mid-twentieth century by a true professional role model of mine, Dr. Albert Ellis. He titled his work Rational Emotive Behavior Therapy[18] and his innovative approach to thinking about thoughts is still used today.[18] A modification of the approach includes three main components: the event that causes the distress, the thoughts about the event, and the resulting feelings.

Take an event in your life that causes distress (e.g., failing a test or receiving negative feedback from a professor or boss) and write it down in column one. Ask yourself how you feel after the event and write down all the negative feelings in column two. Then in column three, ask yourself what your thoughts are during and after the event. For example, "The professor is right; my work is not good at all," "I failed the test and it just means I am not smart like everyone else," or "I am never going to get into college." Be as honest as possible. In column five write how you would like to feel when one of the above events happens. Write down all the ideal feelings you would like to have (e.g., happiness, contentment).

Finally, for column four come back to the thoughts and change them to the exact opposite of what you had in column three. Instead of "The professor is right, I am not good at all," you can change that to, "In this one single incident I may have not done my best work, but I am still okay." What gives you the proof that based on one test, one exam, or one comment you are not capable of performing better the next time? The hope is that the thoughts in column four will lead you to the feelings in column five. Too often we allow our negative thoughts to consume us. We have only so much control over the events in our lives. As for the ones we cannot control, we have choices in how we respond. It is important to pay attention to the many irrational thoughts that might hold us back from living fully. If the thought is not helping you, change it.

If you are a person who sees the glass as half empty, and you believe that everything always happens to you and that whatever happens in your life will lead to failure, then chances are your thoughts frequently become reality. True, negative events will happen, but ask yourself: "Do these events happen all the time, or am I just saying they do?" Ask yourself what proof you have that the conclusion you are assuming will definitely happen. Do not expect defeat. Instead, embrace the possibility of a positive outcome. If the outcome is not to your liking, focus on the learning experience you are able to gain from it.

Gloomy thinkers diminish anything positive that does happen. If you are in school and you fail a test, you have a choice as to how you can respond to that event. You can respond by thinking you are incapable at school work and you are never going to be successful, or you can think about the event as a learning experience. Accept that it is unfortunate, your performance was not so ideal, and experience the feelings associated with those thoughts. Then move forward from that point and find out how you can better yourself in the class and on the next test, thinking about how you would prefer to feel.

If you choose to engage in negative thinking, pay close attention to how and why you think like that. Look deep into your earliest memory as to why you think the way you do and how you can contradict that thought. Additionally, look to role models who think in a more positive way, and make every attempt to understand how they are able to do it. If you do not get it, you have the choice to ask them.

Pay close attention to the fact that you may be focusing on an insignificant problem (e.g., why the line-up at the grocery store is so long, why the airplane is delayed, or why it is raining outside) when in reality there is so much more to focus on that could be a more helpful thought, and which is within your control. For example, waiting in line at the grocery store will take as long as it needs to take — even if it is an extra four minutes, that is okay. Another example is air travel. You do not have control over when the airplane is going to take off, so think about something else while the airlines think about getting you on board when they can. You can be thankful you are not walking to your destination.

Last but not least — if you have difficulty thinking about your thoughts, take a single distressing thought and make a list of all the good things and bad things about that thought. When you see on paper that there are more bad things than good affiliated with the thought, you can choose to now look for an alternative that will help you feel better. Allow for adversity to happen, because it will. Embrace misfortune and take responsibility for the negative thoughts that occur. However, in the moment of negative thinking and feeling, stop yourself, think about whether the thought is helping, and then act on how *you* can make the choice to change it.

So when reflecting on what type of communication properties you want to invest the most time in on your board game, understand the importance of owning all three and how much more well-grounded you can be by building on them, both verbally and nonverbally with yourself and others. Taking time to invest in the thoughts and feelings you are having about certain issues and then communicating them may help you feel at ease when crossing those squares on the board. Liberating yourself of emotional restriction via communication may do more for you than you have ever considered. Pay attention to how often you want to communicate certain feelings and how often you hold back from doing so. If you want to balance the mental and emotional side of your game board, express your thoughts and emotions in any way you know how.

Quick Points

- Verbal expression can release emotion in the hope of hearing, learning, and progressing. Be comfortable expressing yourself verbally regardless of your gender.
- Physical expression can release built-up anger and affiliated negative thoughts and feelings. Inappropriate physical expression may inaccurately attend to the real problem you are facing. Pay attention to the distressing event or why you are choosing to release physical aggression.
- Written expression communicates thoughts, feelings, and emotions that can be revisited on paper to help learn from previous experiences. Use written expression as a reminder of how you have handled negative events in your life before.
- E-mail is a very dangerous form of written expression; send with caution!
- Accept yourself as a valuable person; allow for

negative experiences, but understand you always have choice as to how you can respond to these events to help you feel better about incidents in your life.

Notes Page
Thoughts? Feelings? Intentions? Actions?

_____

_____

_____

_____

_____

_____

_____

_____

_____

_____

_____

_____

_____

_____

_____

_____

_____

_____

_____

_____

_____

_____

CHAPTER 5
Social Balance – Ties Within the Core of the Family Tree

"To the outside world we all grow old. But not to brothers and sisters. We know each other as we always were. We know each other's hearts. We share private family jokes. We remember family feuds and secrets, family griefs and joys. We live outside the touch of time."
~Clara Ortega

ocial behavior is founded on actions, thoughts, feelings, and reactions to society.[19] Social balance involves but is not limited to the right combination of family, friends, significant others, teachers, classmates, fellow employees, and teammates. Regardless of the realm of social activity, I believe the four pillars that may help balance our social lives include: consistency, trust, respect, and honesty. Without those four key elements, you will be establishing social patterns on rocky ground that will eventually lead to disappointment, frustration, and dejection.

Family is the first social network[20] one is exposed to. Therefore, the foundation of who you are, where you come from, and who you aspire to be comes in large part from your family and upbringing. Your family may be the single most important aspect of your social world. The difference between family and friends is that family is forever and friends may come and go. Your family may be both immediate (e.g., parents and siblings) and extended (e.g., aunts, uncles, and cousins) and may also be non-blood members (e.g., close friends or neighbors). It is very common in many religions and cultures to include many people who are not blood related as actual family members.[21] So what is so important about family? Why do you need to care so much about interactions with them?

<u>Dear Parents from Children</u>:

The role that parents play in a child's life can affect how the child will act in the future.[22] The parent needs to ensure the child sees consistency. A child is attentive to more than one is typically aware of. Walter Gretzky, father of the hockey great Wayne Gretzky, was once asked by a parent why it was so important to attend all the Little League games if you cannot even interact with the child throughout the game. His response was that the child feels and appreciates the presence, whether or not the parent is aware of it.

A parent's presence instills in the child's mind that the parent will be in their corner cheering them on both inside and outside the home, and not just when it is convenient. By establishing your presence at their major life events, your children will begin to understand the concepts of support, trust, and consistency. Knowing the parent made the effort will forever be ingrained in their heads, hearts, and minds. If the parent is unable to attend, it is essential the child knows why.

Additionally, it is important that the child does not just hear the explanation, but more so is actively involved in the interaction to ensure understanding. It is important for the parent to conceptualize that prior to preschool, they are the social network[20] for their child. Children will not know of any other forms of active social networks[20] unless you initiate play dates with other children or you are actively involved in their growth and learning. When you decide to have a child and a family of your own, you are taking on the responsibility of a full-time job outside of your place of employment.

Parents today can also fall into three categories: full-time, part-time, or nonexistent. The full-time parent always knows where their children are, is always engaged with them and their activities, and can name their favorite foods and television shows or some of their interests. Then there is the parent who plays the role of uncle or aunt, the parent who shows up for dinner occasionally to eat with the child, the parent who has so little time for the child that every so often they buy the child a present to make the child feel happy and to show love. Although this tactic may work temporarily, it will not sustain itself in the long run.

However, this type of parent is at home so seldom that instead of being a parent they play the role of an uncle or aunt, one who shows up at the house regularly, but the child sees them for a total of only five hours per week. Most often this happens because of priorities with work, and/or fulfilling other interests. Sometimes it is not a choice, as bills have to be paid and one parent's willingness to provide an ideal life for their children may result in them being less present. However, it is important to pay close attention to why a parent may be absent and ensure that the child understands the specific reason(s) as to why that is the case. If parents allow their children to make assumptions or create their own thoughts, this may create a disconnection and thinning family ties.

The third category is the nonexistent parent. The nonexistent parent is one who does not live at home with the child and seems to appear once a year during holidays or birthdays. That is not saying that parents being separated are the difficulty. If you are no longer living with your partner, that does not mean you cannot be actively involved in your child's life. You may be limited to seeing your child only on weekends. That means when it comes time to interacting with your child, you should put away the home office and direct all your attention to him or her. As well, feel free to send your child e-mails or text messages to maintain a connection. If you choose to take on the role of being a parent, be the role, do not just pretend.

Children have to know that you are there for them. Even though you may think they know, how often do you ask them? Of course, there are certain parents who have an arrangement where one parent may live in a different country in order to send money to the family and thus is not present that often. Regardless of the quantity of time spent with children, communicating and embracing in quality time with them will help them better understand your role as the parent and not have to figure it out on their own.

Continuous and consistent interaction with your child will help him or her understand what it means to trust. As children grow up, they may not verbalize how important the little things are, but it helps define who they become. Of course all parents have different degrees of involvement in the lives of their children. The idea is to step back for a moment as a parent and gain a grasp on what type of role you as a parent would like to play, and communicate that with your child to see what their expectations are. The crux of interaction with your children does not come down to the quantity of time spent, but more the quality.

Your child should be able to consistently communicate with you, whether it is verbal[5] or nonverbal.[8] Do not wait for the child to come to you; often they will not do that. Approach your child to know what they are thinking. Remember — they hear everything you say, see everything you do, and they mimic it when the opportunity presents itself. Everything you say and do is learned and retained. Therefore, it is essential to be aware of your words and actions. For example, if you are spending more money than you earn, that is a problem. The child needs to learn that there are limits and that a credit card does not mean free money.

Your role as a parent helps define whom your children will eventually form a social network[20] with and partly how they will behave in social settings. You as the parent decide to live in a certain neighborhood, send your child to a certain school, and enroll them in certain activities within the neighborhood. Once the child is enrolled, it is up to them to create the network. For the first few years of school the social network[20] is created for them. Therefore, where you choose to live, whom you choose to affiliate with, and the school you select for your child can dictate a lot. For example, whom your children will befriend and what types of goals, values, and limits that will be set and attained can be influenced by your choices when it comes to their socialization.

Your job as the parent does not end in the social realm. It is crucial to understand you are not their best friend — you are the parent. Children, and even adults, are always comparing themselves with others, whether it be the food they eat, the clothes they wear, the toys they have, or the way they look. Be aware, know your limitations, understand, but set your parameters.

It is tempting to live vicariously through your children, as they may be engaging in experiences and opportunities you never had. However, the main difference between your childhood and theirs is that they are currently living it, and you already lived yours. You have to be aware of your actions and intentions with respect to what you would like most for your child. You do not have children to account for your childhood regrets. Your children need their own lives, but you cannot remove yourself from their interests! If their interests are similar to yours — great, but if not, you still have to respect, accept, and encourage theirs.

If you grew up playing high school football and your child wants to play chess or enroll in something different like art class, that does not mean they are not living up to your expectations; they are simply forming their own. Your role as a parent emerges when you talk with them about their interests. It is not enough to ask them "How was the game?" "How was school?" and "Are you hungry?" If you ask them short questions, expect shorter answers. Regardless of how old your child is, their answers will be only as deep as your questions. Adolescents tend to share more information with their peers than with their parents.

Too often parents are afraid to broach certain topics with their children, so they choose not to. Avoiding certain topics may give the impression that anything uncomfortable to talk about is forbidden and is thus not shared. The adolescent's response is to turn to their friends. What the child does not understand is that their friends at fifteen may not be their friends at sixteen, whereas their parents will always be there.

Therefore, when the opportunity presents itself for children and parents to speak — take advantage of it. Ask your child open-ended questions[23], such as "What happened in the game today that you enjoyed most?" "What did you study in math class today?" "What activities are you doing in school now that basketball is over?" It seems simple, but it rarely happens. Make it a habit from the early stages of life to actively engage in some form of open communication with your child; it will make for an easier connection later on in life. Quite often, parents will work many hours during the week and have an excellent balance at work and with their husbands/wives or partners and their own friends. However, these same parents may not be able to tell you the name of one of their child's friends. Knowing these types of details may indirectly enhance a connection with the child.

The open exploratory communication a parent has with his or her child will help dictate the degree of consistency, trust, and respect the child has for the parent. For example, if your child chooses to color the speakers with crayons, stop before you react and think how you can be proactive in this scenario. Use challenges as opportunities to grow, learn, and understand *with* — not *at* — your child. Ensure there is an equal balance of attention and interest between the children. If you are unsure whether or not you pay enough attention to one child over another, ask them!

<u>Dear Children from Parents</u>:

So what does that mean for the child? How are you as a child supposed to react and act to create consistency, trust, and respect with your parent(s) and build a mutually exclusive connection? The first thing a child should understand is that parents brought you into this world and grew up during a different generation. However, do not let the age difference define your social connection with your parents. Be aware that they do love you even if they do not show it enough. If they do not show the love you want to receive, try to work on changing that. Both the child and the parent are responsible for a great connection.

The scary thing is that as you grow up, you first believe that your parent(s) or caregivers are like superheroes and that they literally know everything. Moving into your teenage years, you often think they do not know everything; your parents just do not comprehend your generation, and may embarrass you. Oddly enough, as you move into your adult life you may start to realize how much your parents do actually know that goes beyond what a textbook can tell you. It is important to realize this when you are younger so you can truly understand why it is they do what they do when it comes to raising you. If you do not know, ask them.

It is not always about doing the right thing or always saying the right thing. What can help you define trust with your parent(s) or caregivers is a mutual understanding that they can count on you and you can count on them. It is essential to be aware of everything your parents do for you; do not take it for granted. You may think when it comes to providing food, shelter, or money *that's just what parents are supposed to do*. Be that as it may, understand your parent(s)' efforts to do so, and that the toll it takes on them includes obstacles they may hide from you.

Throughout your life your parent(s) and/or caregivers will engage in a variety of activities for you to ensure your happiness and enjoyment in life. It is essential to inform them of how much you appreciate what they do with and for you. In return, your task as the child is to respect their decisions, choices, and values.

The bottom line is that they are trying to make sure you lead a healthy, successful life.

Additional respect lies in the fact that they are older than you and have been through many if not all of the experiences you are going through. Even if you think they do not "get it," they might — and if not, help them to understand; they want to know about your world and what it looks like through your eyes. Respect the fact that they have life experience; look to them for help and opinions, and take the time to listen to what they have to say. Hearing is not enough, as it can be understood as a crescendo of noises. Stop to think for a moment how you obtained the video games you are playing or the iPod you are using. Chances are it was a gift from your parent or another family member.

The least you can do is give them a few minutes of your time — after all, they have given you theirs. They may ask you to do something you do not want to do: mow the lawn, shovel the snow, call your grandmother, or clean your room. Respect their wishes and in turn, chances are they will respect yours.

The game of parent-child relationship is a give and take scenario. It is quite easy as a child only to take, and easy as a parent only to give–but this imbalance might lead to disrespect, frustration, and a strained relationship. The parent and child need to balance their interaction and reliance in order to attain respect, fluidity, and openness.

What can you do to earn their respect? The role of the child is ongoing whether you live with your parents or not. Showing respect for your parents within the home will create a continuous regard for those of the

same category outside the home, extending to teachers, coaches, your friends' parents, etc. To show respect does not necessarily mean to obey orders (even
though it may seem that way). To show respect means
to listen to the values your parents attempt to teach
you and understand not just what they are, but who
they are and what is important about what they are
saying.

Follow the guidelines they set out for you at home
and try to carry that out of the home as well. If guidelines do not exist, set them with your parents. All children will bend and break the rules at some point. No
child can follow all the guidelines and always remain
on track. As a parent, patience and understanding
are required. As a child, an understanding of the point
of the rules is required. It is a team effort. It may help
to not see them as restricting boundaries, but more as
guided options.

Guided options that may help in and out of the
house just for kids:

1. If you take something out, put it back after you
   are done with it.
2. Take responsibility for your choices even if that
   means there will be consequences. After all,
   you are the one who made the choice.
3. If you enter a room and it is clean, make sure
   you leave it the same way it was before you en-
   tered it.
4. Keep your private space (bedroom usually) organized. If you are not an organized person,
   see later chapters on organizational skills.

5. Take care of your siblings.
6. Use the words "please" and "thank you" anytime there is an opportunity to.
7. Eliminate the use of profanity.
8. If you choose to engage in substance use, talk about it with your parents. The simple conversation (although initially uncomfortable) will show your parents that you have enough respect for them to not go behind their backs.
9. Appreciate what you have instead of demanding more. Your parents work very hard at providing everything they can for you; respect that.
10. Give them the time of day; after all, you would not have that day if it were not for them.
11. Listen to what they have to say. If you disagree with it, then talk about it. Closing your ears off is one of the most disrespectful responses from a child.
12. They may be crazy, quirky, and embarrass you often, but they are your parents and that will never change. Be careful as to how you respond when they embarrass you. The fact of the matter is they are who they are and you are not going to change them. Thus, appreciate it and do what you can to make sure you do not become like that, because chances are you will.
13. Ask them how their day was.
14. Ask them if they want to spend some time with you. You don't know how long you will be living in the same city as your parents; therefore take advantage of the time you have before

the time with them becomes restricted to visits.

15. Eat dinner with them. We all lead crazy lives, both parents and children, but taking fifteen minutes away from the insanity that life brings upon us helps contribute to connection and open communication.

16. Show affection (e.g., physical, verbal, or written), but know each parent may like different levels.

17. Talk to them. If you feel they do not understand, help them understand.

18. Minimize your lies. Being truthful will only enhance their respect for you.

19. Treat them the way you would like to be treated.

20. You create the last one ... go ahead.

Your First Roommates

Your siblings bring a different approach to the family dynamic and social balance in your life. Your siblings are to be your partners in crime. All the ruckus and rambunctious behavior that ensues within the home tends to take place between siblings. Creating a strong bond with a sibling is not easy. Sibling connections are to be preached and praised by the parents and grandparents. Initial connections come from play between one another. Children can connect early in life based on both real and imaginary play[24] and especially with siblings. Siblings are the people that you spend the most time with outside of your own peers, because often they live in your room or the one next to you. Therefore, taking advantage of the opportunities you have with your siblings is crucial.

As time moves forward, everyone develops their own individual lives, their own friends, and thus time with siblings decreases, but that does not necessarily mean the connection has to. If a strong foundation has been created with siblings early on, simple maintenance is a lot easier later in life. As that foundation has been created and there is an understanding and respect of each sibling's character, siblings will remain close as long as the effort is put forth.

Establishing and maintaining a strong sibling relationship begins with sharing common toys, games, interests, and sometimes even your bedroom. However, as you grow up, sibling relationships can start to develop on a much deeper level. A strong sibling relationship does not start or sustain itself automatically. Thus, as the older sibling you assume the role of tour guide, showing the younger sibling(s) the ropes, what it is like to be a part of the world, and what you have done so far to succeed.

The younger sibling plays the role of the automatic friend; do not take advantage of this. Simply going across the hall to hang out with, talk to, and interact with your sibling, you can make his or her day! Thus, to establish a strong connection with your sibling(s), interact with them, communicate with them, and show them you care. It does not matter if you are the older sibling or the younger sibling; just showing one another that you care is essential. How do you show you care? Acknowledging birthdays regardless of the age, knowing who their friends are and their interests is essential.

Of course, there comes a time when siblings need to just be with their own friends. However, it is equally important that moments are put aside for siblings to make time for one another outside or conjointly with friends. There are always activities that can be enjoyed together; the key is to make sure that happens.

Common activities that siblings can engage in are games (e.g., video games and board games), watching television around the house, engaging in outdoor activities together, or outings like the movies, the zoo, or sporting events. It is important as a sibling to find that common interest and make time to connect on that level. Distance can separate siblings and will limit their time together. If that is the case, we live in a world where e-mail, long distance phone calls, webcam internet chat sites, and social networking websites are essentially free. So, if face-to-face communication is less likely or less frequent, there are numerous ways to keep lines of communication open to maintain the strong connection.

The most important factor in sibling connection is communication; without it, you are working on a rickety bridge. Therefore, know your siblings, understand their likes and dislikes, understand their behaviors — what makes them happy and what bothers them most. Do not be afraid to ask them questions and give them your thoughts. Again, respect is a key factor in establishing and maintaining a strong sibling connection. Respect your siblings, their time, space, friends, belongings, and thoughts. If you are able to maintain respect for all of the aforementioned and demand the same level of respect in return, you will not overstep your boundaries. You and your siblings will each lead your own independent lives while selecting the moments you choose to share. You will become each other's most comforting and comfortable shoulder on which to lean, if you so choose.

Quick Points

- Parents, talk with your children. They know more than you realize.
- Children, talk with your parents. They know more than you want to admit.
- Be brave and talk about topics that may make you uncomfortable.
- Engage in activities with your siblings. It is okay to be friends with them...really, it is okay.
- Friends will change, but your siblings will not. Communicate your thoughts and feelings with your siblings. Listen, learn, and grow from one another's experiences.

Notes Page
Thoughts? Feelings? Intentions? Actions?

_____

_____

_____

_____

_____

_____

_____

_____

_____

_____

_____

_____

_____

_____

_____

_____

_____

_____

_____

_____

_____

_____

_____

_____

_____

CHAPTER 6

Social Balance – Extending out to the Branches of the Tree

"To the world you may be one person,
but to one person you may be the world."
~Heather Cortez

If you are fortunate enough to grow up with grand-parents in your life, take advantage of it! To establish some form of balance within your family and social life, you need to understand where you came from and where your roots are. Your historical foundation stems beyond your parents to your grandparents.

Your grandparents may seem old to you or less a part of your life than your peers, colleagues, and sig-nificant other. Even though you may not often interact with them, awareness of their influence on your life is vital to understanding where you came from.

Therefore, it is essential to know their history. They grew up in a different time, but never forget that they experienced many of the same things you have and will have, possibly under less than ideal conditions. Most importantly, they have lived through many stages of life that you have yet to reach. They gave and continue to give, while all they want in return is your love and attention, most of the time.

Take the time to speak with them. They will attempt to grasp your perspective, but more than anything, they will feel like they really know their own grandchildren. Call them. They want to hear your voice, and you should want to hear theirs. They look forward to simply hearing the voice of someone they indirectly created and love.

The average grandchild may think that it is not such a big deal to call their grandparents, write them letters or e-mails, or have dinner with them. However, it is important for both of you to gain a better understanding of each other. The lessons learned from grandparents are those that go beyond the textbook — the moments that do not have monetary value, but are in fact invaluable. If you can spend two hours a day searching the internet for random toys on auction sites or three hours chatting online with friends through various internet social networks, chances are you have time to devote to your grandparents — try it.

What can you do to increase communication and connection with your grandparents? Start by attending to some of these steps:

1. Call them routinely; they want to hear from you. Often, all it takes is a five-minute conversation. They just want to hear your voice. There is always time for a short phone call, and there is a lot of feeling in hearing someone's voice.

2. Go out for dinner with them every so often. I know it may not be as fun as dinner with your friends, or it may not be the coolest thing to do, but your friends will wait. Your grandparents deserve to take priority.

3. Visit with them at family functions. Take a moment to listen to them and hear what they have to say. You never know what you might learn.

4. Go on a date with them. They are not incapable of enjoying life. You will only further enhance their life by sharing your youth and energy with them. Find out what they like to do in their spare time and do that with them. Make it a monthly occurrence.

5. Be aware of their age and mannerisms. They may have little quirks about them that bother you, but you cannot let that hold you back from interacting with them. Understand that they are your past, present, and future as they help define where you came from, who you are, and where you are going. If you do not understand that, take the time to try to find out. They are a strong source of historical information. As you slowly find out where you're going in life, it is essential to understand where you came from.

It is also important to try and connect with your parents' siblings, your aunts and uncles. Of course every family is different in its size, structure, and geographical location, but be aware of how many uncles and aunts you do have and take the time to acknowledge that they exist. Your aunts and uncles are extensions of your parents. These people share many similarities and differences with your parents. They present an alternative perspective on life. They grew up in a similar point in time as your parents did, but bring a varying light to the topic of life experience.

Do not discount their advice regardless of their age. Pay attention to them and attempt to understand their perspective on life; you never know what you might learn from them. Just because they are not your parents does not mean you cannot talk to them about similar issues. After all, they may bring forth a perspective that perhaps your parents did not think of or could just not relate to. Take advantage of the fact that you have additional sets of parental figures.

The wonderful thing about having aunts and uncles is there is a high chance they may have children and thus generate cousins for you. The age gap from your oldest cousin to your youngest may vary greatly. However, the age gap between cousins does not necessarily dictate your level of closeness to one another. You may be just as connected with a cousin who is ten years older than you the same way you are connected with a cousin who is ten days older than you. Regardless of the age gap, you decide how close you want to be with your cousins. Cousins can play a significant role in your life, as they are part of your generation. Even if they do not live in the same city as you, communicate with your cousins in other ways. Take time to get to know them. You may find you have more in common than you realize.

Family is an automatic bond, a bond that can be broken only if you choose to break it. As you know, there are so many different family members out there with different connections, differing socializing patterns, different personalities, different interests, and different beliefs. However, they are still family, and whether you like it or not, they will always be related to you. Thus, it is important to connect with them on all levels, from the grandparents to the cousins, and everything in between.

Your family is like a bag of mixed nuts. There are similar nuts in the bag, and groups or even categories of nuts, but no two nuts are exactly the same. Some nuts are more expensive than others, some are sweeter than others, some have different shapes and sizes, and some are just there in their purest form. It is up to you whether you choose to attend to and/or like some or the entire bag you have been given.

Communicate with them. Send e-mails, add them on your internet social networking sites, call them, write to them, text message them, visit them, and spend the time to figure out who they are. If verbal[15] or written[17] communication is not your strength, then use your strengths to gain a better relationship with your family. Perhaps it may be more comfortable for you to paint them a picture, take them ice skating, go see a movie — anything to establish a bond. The most important part about connecting with family members is doing it more than once.

Connecting with different family members is nice, but has staying power only if you repeat the performance. You do not want to end up saying "I already went there for dinner" when in fact three years have already gone by since then. Think about the last time you interacted with a family member and if either of you has celebrated a birthday in the interim. You do have the opportunity to recognize all special occasions of a family member. It is a good excuse and reminder to keep in touch. Know that friends will come and go, but family is forever.

As you pass the family square on your board game, pay attention to why you feel it is important to attend to the individuals that make up that square. If it is important to own that square, remind yourself why, think about it, and act on it. Call your family members, write to them, but remember they all fulfill different needs at different times in your life. So, attend to when and how you will integrate your family into balancing an aspect of your social world. Instead of being intimidated to land on that square, embrace it and appreciate the events that come with it, good and bad.

Quick Points

- Appreciate that your family extends beyond your parents and siblings.
- Appreciate your grandparents, aunts, and uncles—call them now.
- Laugh, cry, and smile with your cousins even if

you have only met them once.
- Share your thoughts with your cousins. Chances are they have had or will have similar experiences.
- Connect with the elderly; they can provide you with insight that you cannot obtain from academics or any professional setting.

Notes Page
Thoughts? Feelings? Intentions? Actions?

_____

_____

_____

_____

_____

_____

_____

_____

_____

_____

_____

_____

_____

_____

_____

_____

_____

_____

_____

_____

_____

CHAPTER 7
It's a Jungle out There: The Powerful Influence of Friendships

*"We are so often caught up in our destination that
we forget to appreciate the journey, especially the
goodness of the people we meet on the way."*
~Author Unknown

S ocial patterns[20] are often dictated by the society in which you live. However, on a more direct scale, how you choose to act on these patterns is significantly dictated by your peers, (i.e., the people you see or communicate with most often aside from your immediate family). Even though Hollywood or New York may set the standards for "what's cool," the stars in Hollywood are not the people your typical day revolves around. It is the people with whom you interact with every day that help define who you are; you are not so much defined by someone you see on TV or in a movie. It is in part the social relationships that help you form connections and understanding of who people are and how that meshes with your true self.

As you will find out or may have already found out, there is nothing smooth about socialization in Western society. There are various elements you should be aware of to create some form of social balance in your life and thus diminish the stress, fear, and frustration that emerge from social anxiety.[25] This discussion on socialization and its effect on your overall life balance will start from the outside and move inward.

From the outside, what you wear is dictated by the fashion trends of a society. In our superficial society we often judge people on a first impression. We look at what they are wearing and how they put themselves together. There is the old question of if you saw a man wearing ragged clothing and untidy hair versus a man wearing a suit and tie with polished shoes and coiffed hair and both asked to borrow a dollar, who would you be more inclined to give the money to? Your level of comfort may be increased with someone who is better-kept. The same holds true when meeting new people, developing friendships, or looking for a significant other. The bottom line is it has to start somewhere, and that is usually with the clothing, from the outside in.

It starts from the shoes up to the hat (if necessary). What do you see first? When you are a child, if the person next to you has the same color socks and also likes apples, you automatically become friends. In your teens, it is someone who sports certain cultural trends or the most hip attire. In your twenties, it may be the person who wears the nice suit and does so with confidence or has similar career aspirations. I have noticed that many people feel the message is such that the clothes and the physical features on the outside initially create some form of interest. Pay attention: that very message is just a collection of thoughts, when in fact there may not be evidence.

We are all looking for someone as close as possible to ourselves based on their attire, when in reality we are wearing what we are told to wear. We are selecting clothes that the merchants place on the shelves, which designers have labeled as "in," or mere fads based on what is advertised by celebrities. Therefore, it is important to pay attention and realize what it is that makes us believe we are choosing our own attire. The reality is we are not making independent decisions about our attire, as much as we think. We are selecting from the options created by the industry and not what necessarily makes us feel most comfortable. As a result we miss the boat on individualizing our attire and become part of the masses.

What ends up happening is we spend hundreds or even thousands of dollars on articles of clothing, all to ensure that we "fit in" with clothes we may not even "fit into." When in reality all we may want to do is go home and wear what is most comfortable — sweat pants and a t-shirt. If that is the case, then do it! Do not hold back your desire for comfort. If you are most comfortable in what you are wearing, you will feel more comfortable in how you act.

Of course, this does not hold true for the working world and you cannot usually get away with wearing what is most comfortable. However, you can still look dressy without having to sacrifice comfort and style ... and hundreds of dollars. Ensure that what you wear fits right on the outside and in turn on the inside. If you are confident in your own opinion and choices, then pick the clothes that will define who you are. Pick the clothes that feel best for you, and not because of a certain celebrity or an advertisement you see on television, the internet, or a billboard. You are your own person; let your clothes help define that.

In selecting various clothes and certain brand names you may pay more for either higher quality or simply a higher-end designer. The reality is you can find a look that suits you without breaking your bank. The fact of the matter is the clothes are simply just the initial spotlight that will lead you into a more in-depth conversation. Thus, being properly attired does play a role in first impressions. This importance is not to be discounted as purposeless and purely materialistic. In fact, there is much more that clothing can do for you than simply clothe you.

Do not let the clothes define who you are, but more so how you feel. Let yourself define who you are and use the clothing as your accent. Realize though that attire will change from setting to setting. What you wear at school may not be so acceptable at a job, a wedding, or a bar mitzvah. Be aware of social norms while accounting for your comfort, your style, and your culture. Over and above it all, remember that confidence is not only always in fashion, it plays an important role in how you wear your clothes, which is more important in a first impression than what you wear. Confidence will define your posture, your body language, your assertiveness, and your happiness, which are all related to attractiveness.

Choose what you feel is most age-appropriate and situation-specific, and what you think will make you feel better, but be aware of the cost-effective ratio. Lastly, much like everything else in life, new experiences start off with a spike and then eventually plateau. The same holds true for the new friend selection process. You start off with an initial spark and then eventually with more communication and interaction, the friendship plateaus with various peaks and valleys. Based on the superficial society we live in, that initial spark or first step is often determined by how you present yourself.

Compared to the family, friends are the people you choose to love forever or choose to love for the time being. Friends make up a significant portion of your social life, and in turn a lot of your social preferences and choices. The concept of friends can be written about in volumes and volumes of books, journals, and various other literary forms. To help create the social balance among friends it is important to emphasize what defines a friend, the socialization patterns affiliated with friends, and the people you choose to affiliate with.

Regardless of how old you are, you are always making new friends, forming new impressions on others, and continuously re-establishing yourself. If we could all have the same friends from kindergarten, life would be so simple. However, even if we did have the same friends from when we were three apples high, chances are we would not be very happy with ourselves. We experience a lot of growth as soon as we start riding a bicycle; it is important to embrace it. We change so much as individuals — as do our careers, interests, and choices. Therefore, it is essential to continuously make new connections that parallel these changes. New friends enable us to move forward and learn about ourselves, because chances are the interests we shared at three years old are no longer the same at this point in our lives. Therefore, as we change as people, we change our immediate social circles.

As teenagers, we all feel a need to fit in, both into the right clothes and the right social circles. When the commercials, after-school specials, and classroom lectures talk about the difficulties of being a teen, there is some merit to what they are saying. However, the teen tornado you are warned about is only as bad as you make it. There is this false assumption that at midnight on your thirteenth birthday you will automatically change into a freewheeling, drug-crazed, disrespectful, nicotine-smoking, loud-music-playing rebel without a cause. Sorry to say, that is not so much the case. Teenage years are another developmental process that happens over time, with choice, and not in an instant.

The emergence of teenage stardom all boils down to the concept of choice. You make all your own choices and you participate in all your own activities. No one will hold you down with a lighter to your face and say you have to smoke this cigarette or you have to take a hit from the bong. Most teens will eventually be presented with many choices as they go through junior high, high school, and part of college. The key is what you as a teen decide when you are faced with these choices, or what you as the parent teach your teen about choices. Your choices emerge from a recurring life theme of confidence. Those who are more confident will make their own choices and may not succumb to peer pressure.[26]

So, how can you build your confidence, and in turn choose the option that directs you away from danger? Start with something you are good at and work on it until you plateau; then pick something else while maintaining participation in the first interest. For example, if you are talented at playing the violin and you play five times a week, play the violin until you feel quite confident in your abilities, then diminish your time devoted to it so you can add a new activity into your life (e.g., creative writing, reading, or athletics). Begin the new activity by practicing two or three times a week. Set aside a certain amount of time per week for the new activity and work on it to see if you enjoy it. If you enjoy it, then keep going. Then add a third activity to the list and so on and so forth, all the while not deserting your previous talents.

You will be a multi-dimensional person, and you will offer a lot to the social world. Even the greatest athletes and musicians out there do not excel at just one activity. Develop many interests and appeal to many different groups of people, all the while choosing activities that you like. Understand, though, that you can always improve — but only in the activities you feel you want to. Understand that you can be as good as you want to be. These activities help you identify your interests and expand your social connections. Thus participate, attempt, enjoy — and in turn, you will begin to build your confidence in those areas.

Self-esteem is the appreciation of one's worth and importance in society.[27] Often, having a lot of confidence means a high level of self-esteem, but just because they may be related, it does not necessarily mean that one leads to the other. Just because one has confidence does not guarantee they will feel good about themselves. A simple way of looking at how much you like yourself is standing in front of the mirror, liking what you see, and how you feel about what you see (without distorting your image, both figuratively and literally). The more you like about what you see, the more able and willing you may be to put yourself out there in the public eye. It is easier said than done. The bottom line is to establish a level of self-esteem[27] that allows you to be confident enough to make your own choices as opposed to having them made for you by others.

Common self-esteem issues are body weight and shape, height, hair color, skin type, and academic performance.[27] Make yourself aware of what is negatively affecting your self-esteem the most, and change it. Understand that everyone is good at something, and everyone can succeed at something.

You may be reading this and thinking you are not good at anything, or you are just average. Pay attention closely here: you believe only what you *choose* to believe. So, in comparison to the people around you, you may not be as tall, or you may not have the desired measurements, but your body is not what should dictate how you feel. If you believe you are not as good as the others around you, you will carry yourself that way. As a teenager and individual in your twenties, thirties, and beyond no one is there to pick you up off your feet and get you to change your attitude. You may have strong support from family members or friends, but they cannot get inside your mind and change your thought process. You are the only one who can do that: own the responsibility.

Again, it all begins with self-esteem[27], and the ability to raise that level so that you like what you see and what you feel. Be prepared for failed attempts. Just because you fail does not mean you are incapable of success. You just have to find your own talent and allow yourself to become comfortable with strange new situations.

Failure happens throughout life; it puts things into perspective for us. Sometimes we have to experience the failure to really understand and value what it feels like, and move forward from there. If we do not succeed at a task, we have to go back to the drawing board, reevaluate, and understand how we can improve. The same holds true for friendships. Sometimes in our lives we have to make the choice as to which kind of friendships we want to keep, which we want to create, and which we no longer connect with.

As you continue to grow, chances are you will move from city to city (especially during your twenties), continuously establishing new friends in the belief that at all costs you must hang on to old superfluous friendships or establish numerous new ones. Furthermore, the same applies to people who become friends with new people within the same city. However, over time they may realize they just do not want to invest the effort in maintaining the connection as priorities shift. It is okay to change your friends. If you choose to be friends only with the people you first met when you opened your eyes to this world, you may be missing a whole variety of people.

The reality is that the world can be your best friend, but that does not mean you have to be best friends with the world. You may prefer that, but it is not a must. Thus, there comes a point in every person's life when they just have to be honest and say: "Who do I want my real friends to be?" or "Who do I connect with the most and who do I want as acquaintances?" As we grow up from childhood to adulthood, we evolve from having the best friends ... to the right friends. I am not saying you need to be rude, disgraceful, or malicious, and cut off ties with friends you no longer connect with. It is just important that you are honest with yourself and the parties involved.

Ask yourself, "What exactly is it that I am hanging on to?" If you are hanging on to something, know the reason why. If the reasons are not good enough for you, then be okay making a choice that will help your thoughts, feelings, body, and mind. The bottom line is that a cost-benefit analysis needs to be done. If you realize that a friendship costs you more time and creates additional negative emotions, stress, and distractions than the benefits received, it is okay to diminish the connection. You have your own life to live and cannot let others direct it by their preferences, your life...your choice. Do not forget, though, it is a two-way street and you could be on the receiving end of it. Accept it and learn from the experience.

You spend much of your teens and twenties in practice, preparing you for the world in which you will eventually play a more permanent role, for example parenting or career. Thus, if you fail, all you can do is go back and try again. If you gave up on everything you have tried once, you would be missing a lot that life has to offer. The positive side of failure is to know that there is always another chance. In this case, it is the grueling social scene of teenage years that can overwhelm people. You have to be willing to take the risk, take the chance, and if all else fails, try again using a different technique.

What is the worst that could happen if you approach a group of potential peers and they laugh at you because of what you said, or one of them makes a comment about your clothes? If they are that superficial, chances are you do not want them as friends anyway. Another strategy is to talk with just one person from the group. It is a lot easier to deal with one person than go in single-handed and attempt to talk to five. Complying with the tendencies of your social world is an unfortunate reality among teens. One may adjust to the general attitude of the group for approval, when in fact he or she may not actually be revealing their honest opinion or preference.[26] So, approach the individual as opposed to the group, and develop a real and honest relationship that will be stronger than the alternative.

You can practice by spending less time in front of a screen and more time approaching random people at stores, in the park, or even at your school. Ask them a simple question, such as how they are doing, but be sure to listen for an answer. Alternatively, you can compliment them, perhaps on their attire. Regardless of the topic, you will learn how to approach and how to respond to a new interaction. Build that confidence up to allow yourself the freedom to approach anyone without hesitation or worry about what they will think. Once you have that self-esteem within, how you approach, your social scene can be limitless.

Your attitude, opinion, and confidence will be forever changing as you continue to roll the dice on your board game. The hope is that the one thing that remains a constant is being true to yourself and the friendships you seek, build, and sustain each time you decide to invest in one of the social properties of friends. I have followed the simple words of my friend, Shona, who once said: "Treat people the way you would like to be treated [see the poem "*I am*" at the end of the chapter] and the way they would like to be treated." Those words in their purest form promote building a friendship on respect, honesty, and simplicity in the hope of reciprocation.

Keep your approach and thoughts simple and natural. But never forget that friendships will change and the importance of certain friends will also change. Each time you circle your game board of life, understand that you may invest different amounts of time at different phases of your life. So, pay close attention to why you are making certain friendships when you are. If it is difficult to establish connections, try to realize you can own that property if you put forth the effort to.

I am ...

I am a caring girl who likes to be with friends.
I wonder if my friends now will be my friends forever.
I hear music in the sky.
I see myself rollerblading along the beach. I want to
make a difference in the world.
I am a caring girl who likes to be with friends.

***

I pretend to be a professional artist.
I feel wet paint drying on my hands.
I touch my multicolored beads. I worry about the
environment.
I cry when my friends cry.
I am a caring girl who likes to be with friends.

***

I understand that nobody lives forever.
I say: treat people the way you would like to be
treated.
I dream that I climb mountains.
I try to do my very best in school.
I hope the world will be at peace.
I am a caring girl who likes to be with friends.

***

~Shona Goorvich~

Quick Points

- Choose your own style. What you wear can be your choice.
- Be open to meeting new friends all the time. You never know how they may change your perspective.
- When substance use enters your social world, pay attention to what choices you are making and why.
- Stay true to yourself when you are with your friends, and live in the moment.
- Do not complicate your social world. If social plans become stressful, step back and ask yourself why. Keep it simple and enjoy.

Notes Page
Thoughts? Feelings? Intentions? Actions?

_____

_____

_____

_____

_____

_____

_____

_____

_____

_____

_____

_____

_____

_____

_____

_____

_____

_____

_____

_____

_____

_____

_____

CHAPTER 8
Dating...Winning a Game You Choose to Play

"Looking back on our lives, we notice that our biggest growth spurts have been the direct result of overcoming our greatest challenges. Heartbreak; troubling relationships, loneliness and the like are offered to us not as "yet another opportunity to suffer," but as opportunity for promotion to color-fast fulfillment."
~Will Dalton

It is important to acknowledge that in the dating world every relationship will look different. Therefore, it is essential to be aware of and sensitive to the abundant differences that exist in our world and embrace each and every one of them regardless of what your preference is. We live in a very diverse world and it is imperative you keep your eyes open to these differences.[21] If a certain type of relationship or prefer-ence works for one person and does not work for you, that is their choice, not yours. It is important to be open and sensitive to all types of relationships and the cul-tural differences within and between.[21]

Therefore, when reading this chapter on dating, understand that there may be some generalizations that fit and some that do not fit with your experience. However, after interacting with hundreds of high school and college students across the country over the years, I figured I would summarize the tendencies I noticed throughout. Additionally, I will highlight what to be aware of when entering the dating world to help balance a section of your social row on the board game of your life.

I see three phases of dating in life regardless of your sexual orientation.[28] Phase one is dating to enjoy the company of another individual who is more than a friend. You are not thinking about spending the rest of your life with the person. You are dating to have a good time and learn what you do not want or do not prefer. The second phase is that of dating to be in a relationship (more long-term). You see the person you are with or the person you seek as someone with whom you want to spend a lot of time and can see it lasting more than a few weeks or a few months.

There is depth to the person and your connection that goes beyond initial attraction (physical and/or mental). The relationship becomes a significant part of each other's lives. You formulate a unique connection of understanding that goes beyond the surface. The long-term relationship can be anything from months to years. The bottom line is that you think about the person before you go to bed, when you wake up in the morning, and much of your time is spent either with the person or at the very least caring for the person much more than the average close friend.

Finally, phase three transpires. You have just come from a long-term relationship or you have dated for a while and you have grown quite a bit since then. Thus, in this phase, you find you are looking for permanence with this partner. You imagine how a family may look and a future with that someone special. If you are not currently with the person who brings you into this phase, you are at a place where you know everything you do not want out of a relationship and you have a clear idea of exactly what you do want. You have hit phase three: dating for permanence.

Permanence with a partner may look different for everyone: common law, cohabitants, or marriage. Nevertheless, while others may think differently, a permanent partner is seen as a non-refundable transaction. Even though everything in society has some sort of refund policy, the permanent partner is one thing that is preferred to be forever; 'til death do you part. You are at the point where you know what the pillars are that help define a strong relationship (in your mind) that could last forever, and at this point you set out to find that.

Your priorities of the dating continuum shift as you progress from phase one through to phase three. For example, physical attractiveness may not be number one, it may be number seven or eight on your list of essential qualities in a partner. Conversely, similar ideals with respect to how you want to live your life may be number one or two, whereas when you were dating to date it was nine or ten on the list of priorities.

When dating, it is imperative to expect that you are put on a pedestal by your partner, and your partner should expect the same thing in return. You may not care or be comfortable with being placed in such high regard, but expect it and settle for nothing less. If you settle for someone who does not place you at this level, call that into question. They are the person you should be able to trust. In good times and bad, your partner should be in your corner through all your ups and downs. Through sickness and in health, that person will be there, and if not, their dedication to you should be brought into question.

I will not define love, as I believe everyone has their own definition and expectations. One significant requirement, however, is that you both need and want each other's presence in each other's lives. Moreover, it is a need that is not just some of the time, but at all times in all ways: physically, emotionally, and mentally. The way in which you communicate that love may be different, but it is to be synchronized. This can and will look different for all folks.

What is it that women want? What is it about males that creates such a strong desire for women and men to be attracted to some and not others? During adolescence and beyond, females tend to seek partners who can be gentle, emotional, and have the ability to invest in the relationship, with the physical desires emerging during late adolescence and into the twenties.[29] Depending on your sexual orientation[28], it is the nice, shy, quiet people who often have respect for the women, but lack the confidence to approach them or do not want to interfere with someone else they may already be interested in. So it is not so much the nice folks that finish last, it is the less assertive that may lose out while the more assertive and more confident folks often come out ahead of the game. Assertiveness does not imply rudeness.[30]

Treating a woman with respect is essential to understand when you are younger. Most will realize later in life that the nice person is who they want to finish first. Women in their teens sometimes seek one or two attributes — funny, caring, tough, athletic, fashionable, or smart — but by no means will they seek out all of the above. Often, what women seem to want are people like themselves. Therefore, if you are a female interested in athletics, humor, and socializing, you will seek someone similar to you. If you are a female who is primarily occupied by substance abuse, roaming the streets at night with your peers, and some defiance, then you may seek that.

Last, but definitely not least — without you even realizing it, women in their teens and beyond want to be stimulated and complimented in any way, shape, or form (as many of us do to some extent). That is not saying the only thing they want is intimacy, because that is far from true. What they do seem to want, without their partner thinking they want it, is someone who will be different, someone who will assert themselves[30], while protecting, and someone who will not be afraid of trying new things. They tend to seek someone who will be there to compliment them, raise their self-esteem, and increase their confidence.

They may present themselves as shy, quiet young females, but really they are more mature than most males[29] and are more ready for certain curiosities sooner than their partner may be. The difference is that they may be able to control their urges far more readily than male partners. Take for example a person who may wear their thoughts on their shorts. I know some people out there think that is not the case and they do not want to offend certain women. So what happens is that they step back and someone takes over. Then where does the less assertive one finish? Well, it sure is not first.

The female can be a very precious and delicate individual. However, as they may be the most sensitive during high school or even earlier, they may stab (not literally) their friends in the back over and over again if it means they get the partner they want. It is a violent aspect of the social scene, but it is all part of the game, and all genders play the role quite well. The bottom line is most of the relationships that take place in high school may not last beyond receipt of the diploma, especially with so many people relocating so often.

Now the male, on the other hand, seems to be a lot less difficult to grasp. What qualities seem to be of most intriguing to the male during high school can be inferred with your own imagination, depending on your preferences. It is that simple. Sure, they want a partner who will be by their side during their activities or interests, but for the most part the guy wants the partner to be mature, developed, and come with the least amount of baggage possible. Many guys seem to feel it is impossible to find a person without some sort of issues or concerns. Gentlemen, do not think the same does not hold true for your gender. Many believe the same is true when seeking men. It is natural — we all have baggage, both males and females — but the difference between the male form and female form is that males tend to be less emotionally involved in the baggage that they hold, or simply hold it back or express it differently.[31]

Therefore, when it comes to the males in high school the tendency (which does not necessarily have to be the norm) is that they tend to want one thing – action. Again, note this is a tendency, but is not necessarily the case with every male. They may choose not to admit it, they may choose not to reveal it, but they are undoubtedly thinking about it. Now of course the individual who is more willing to be aggressive or assertive in this realm is favored by most males to a certain degree. How you present yourself and your intentions is, above all, your choice. Be sure, though, that you are staying true to yourself to help prevent unwanted circumstances.

It is important to pay close attention to why males, females, and transgender individuals dress a certain way. It is imperative to realize that you can be attractive while still staying clothed. We live in a very sexualized culture where music videos advertise that dressing half-naked will land you the partner you desire — however, that is often not the case in the long run. Again, it is important to be true to yourself and not dress in a certain way that influences a character you are not trying to be.

The bottom line is that regardless of your preference and what males, females, or transgender individuals want, being most comfortable with you is what seems to be most important. If that means you have to alter your image slightly, then adapt accordingly. Remaining in touch with your core self will help keep you balanced regardless of the opinions from others.

Nevertheless, males seem to be less complex and just want the *action*. Of course that will vary and the definition of "action" will change as they get older, from holding hands, to kissing, certain caressing, and then of course intimate relations. However, physical contact is just one aspect of the relationship, and the average male still wants to be cared for, respected, and treated with honesty and integrity. Keep in mind it also depends on the social status of his male friends at that time. If all his peers are in relationships, most males will do anything to be a part of that, even if for only a few weeks.

The difference with some males and their relationship tendencies is they may invest less effort because something better may come along, and will end a relationship without even thinking about it.[29] Males seem to be less attached unless they are with someone who can offer them everything they desire. The males who are more into dubious acts, crass behavior, and various substances will seek partners similar to that nature. Moreover, those males who are kind-hearted, sincere, honest, and trustworthy tend to be seeking partners of that same nature.[29] Now of course there are exceptions to that.

The kind-hearted male who seeks excitement or

thrill in a more spontaneous partner, or the rugged, tough, hard core punk will seek the sweet, kind-hearted, trusting individual. What has to be looked at in that case is why those males seek those types of partners. Refer back to Chapter Four on emotional and mental balance to gain a better understanding of why you think and feel what you do, and how that can impact your dating world.

Often, the males looking for some spontaneity have not really had much in their lives and feel they can get there with someone who will push them. Moreover, those crash and bang tactless males somewhere deep inside are actually caring, considerate, and compassionate individuals who may act a certain way because of social pressure.[26] Either way, whichever male you are, you are to understand you are responsible for all your own choices. If you choose to seek out certain partners, understand that it may not last and he or she may not be the one you want to spend the rest of your life with. Finally, whether you are twenty-eight, twenty-three, sixteen, or thirteen there is plenty of time for plenty of choices; just be sure you are the one who is involved in making them.

Relationships and the Tennis Court

You have always known how to play tennis. When you play with certain friends you do your regular thing as you have for years, but after a while it becomes that same old thing. The game is still fun, but your energy and enthusiasm for the sport plateaus. However, every so often someone comes along and forces you to elevate your game. You are not changing your strokes, or your skill; you are just that much more engaged in the game and more willing to rise to the occasion. You enjoy the powerful and revitalizing rallies, and the challenge comes through in your passion for the game. You are then forced to send and receive some shots from different angles with more precision and power.

When it is all said and done, you know you still love to play tennis, and enjoy it that much more when someone on the other side of the net hits the ball back with the same zest as you do. Therefore, try new things and meet new people. At some point, you will find the partner who makes you try harder, increases your enthusiasm and excitement, teaches you new skills, and challenges you overall.

It is important to be honest with yourself and with the person whom you choose to date, to be sure you are communicating exactly what you are thinking and feeling. Reveal these thoughts and feelings in your actions even if it hurts sometimes. See new people all the time, meet new people all the time, go on dates without thinking of the ramifications of the relationship extending for years or what others may think. For all you know it could end after you say good night, or it could go on for years.

As we all know, you do not reach the Super Bowl or the Stanley Cup after one game. Very rarely will you win the World Series after one game, and therefore you have to take some wins and losses before you get there. Moreover, once you reach the cup finals it takes some time and some wins and losses to finally get your cup. We try out different relationships, take some wins take some losses, and do not establish permanence with the first person we date, as they may be early round upsets to learn from (e.g., in high school or college). Eventually you find the match that feels as if you have reached the cup, the silver dream.

You play out the series with all your heart and after some time you say to yourself: "I got it. I have found and reached my quest for the silver dream!" Once you get there and you have met that natural connection, do not let it go! If someone fumbles and you fall out of first place as a relationship ends, perhaps it is for the best. The worst thing you can do is get angry; the best thing you can do is accept it and appreciate the journey — chances are you have both gained a lot from each other. Do not pretend the person loses their significance in your life. They just hold a different place in your heart as you continue to progress and better understand yourself and your world.

It is okay if relationships do not work out. They are not to be seen as failures, but more so as learned and lived experiences. If you do not experience these setbacks, how will you cope with them if and when they happen later in life? When you are in a relationship, you spend a lot of time trying to get to know someone else. When a relationship does not work out, one of the hardest parts of being single is learning to know yourself. Before anyone can complement you as a partner, it is important you best understand yourself. That way, when a relationship begins, the person truly receives all of you as a whole person, and not someone with unresolved thoughts, feelings, and emotions who chooses to be distant.

Once you have met your match, the one who will challenge you, connect with you, and force you to elevate your natural ability to be there when you are needed the most, you've got it – a life partner. Allow friends to introduce you to potential partners, as most relationships begin that way.[29] Enjoy your teens and twenties dating, seeking, and better understanding yourself and the people you seek as significant others. Allowing for the time to seek new experiences will allow you to better understand yourself and what you want. Just be sure to know what you want. My friend Lee said it best: When seeking a significant other, you need to ask yourself if you want a partner or a project.

Therefore, when you find that partner, you will be ready when your championship presents itself — or when what the board game refers to as an *opportunity* approaches — sometimes without you even realizing it. Revisiting the board game, you can see that self-confidence[32] immediately follows significant others. The reason is because how you feel about yourself and your ability can influence how you approach others romantically. Additionally, it is important to be aware of how important both properties are to attaining a social balance in your life.

Quick Points

- Trust, respect, and honesty are three essential components that cannot be taken for granted;

nor are they automatic or equivalent.

- Communication ... communication ... communication: embrace all forms of it throughout any relationship, always!
- Listen to your gut. It often speaks the loudest.
- Ensure that you your mind, body, heart, and soul are all talking to each other.
- Tell the significant people in your life that you appreciate them, and why.

Notes Page
Thoughts? Feelings? Intentions? Actions?

CHAPTER 9
Social Balance: The Local Street Pharmacy of Social Circles

"Nobody grows old merely by living a number of years. We grow old by deserting our ideals. Years may wrinkle the skin, but to give up enthusiasm wrinkles the soul."
~Samuel Ullman

The third major aspect of socialization in your teens (and unfortunately your twenties and sometimes thirties and beyond) is that of drugs and behavior. Of course we could not go through the social balance on the board game of life without passing the illustrious square of substance abuse. Fittingly, the substance abuse square lies amidst self-confidence, self-esteem[27], and opportunities. It is not a matter of whether or not you will have the opportunity to be surrounded by drugs and alcohol. It is a question of when, which drugs, what type of alcohol, and the choices you make when these situations present themselves. How do you balance all the pressures that come your way and still remain true to yourself? As hard as society tries to diminish the substance use and abuse problem, drugs, alcohol, and cigarettes are available at the most curious stage of life, teenage years. However, it is possible to manage the continuous flow of substance use without socially isolating yourself.

Regardless of which high school or college you attend and in which city you live, alcohol, drugs, and cigarette smoking will be made available, often without you even realizing it. Additionally, the aforementioned substances may be more readily available than a bag of carrots. Much like many other life experiences, it comes down to choice. It may come easy for certain people to be smart, successful students or professionals, but even smart people can make dumb choices.

During junior high, high school, and college the common drugs available tend to be marijuana, mushrooms (better known as 'shrooms), Ecstasy, and even cocaine and crystal methamphetamine, often referred to as "meth." Of course the latter two are not as common until later once the original *supposed* high of marijuana is no longer enough; nevertheless, they need to be mentioned. Just because some of these substances are available does not mean they need to be part of life.

Of course not every single junior high, high school, or college in North America has a problem with the substances mentioned above. However, when the media discusses the war on drugs in the high school systems and colleges, they are doing so in part to create awareness; by no means do they intend you to try them. If some of the aforementioned substances are part of your school's culture, then pay very close attention as to why one might choose to engage in such acts.

Regardless of the drug options available to you, they often guide the various social circles as you progress through your teens. There are the groups that have tried various substances, there are the groups that do it on weekends or occasionally, and then there are the groups that have replaced their level of oxygen with various intoxicants. In spite of the groups out there, you yourself are making a choice to either be with or against the drug options. Often, one will choose to become a part of the drug community to fit in, just to be affiliated with something. However, as discussed in Chapter Eight, there are much healthier and substantial alternatives to fitting in and making friends.

Drugs provide an escape from reality.[33] Those who choose to integrate themselves with drug-induced people tend to be running from something, momentarily escaping reality. Ask yourself, what is attracting you to drugs. Curiosity may play a large role, especially in your teens, but that goes only so far. Once you have tried it, the curiosity no longer exists. If you choose to go beyond the curiosity, it is essential to examine what is attracting you to these substances. Refer to the chapter on verbal, physical, and written expression to help you explore the source of the attraction and your thoughts.

During adolescence you are faced with new unforeseen stress, pressure, and change. It is easier to avoid than confront. So, some take the easy path and chose to avoid because they feel the need to "do what everyone else is doing." Thus, they use an illegal substance to escape temporarily from their world. Why? Because it will take them to a place that seems to be worry-free. However, as Sir Isaac Newton discovered, What goes up must come down, and coming down is a much more painful experience than dealing with the issue at hand. If you are running from some form of stress or fear, your high will last only so long before you eventually plunge down and have to face the same inevitable reality that you attempted to avoid. The only other result of drug use is never to face this inevitable reality you have been avoiding — otherwise known as death.

However, what happens when that high just becomes boring? Before you know it, you have dropped all your interests and all you want to do is find those friends who will do it with you. However, the drugs will also slow down your heart rate, mental processing, and your short-term memory.[33] As a result, you may lose interest in your everyday activities like athletics, school, work — and most importantly, the friends who did not choose to ride with you on your magic carpet.

As your productivity declines you will become easily agitated because of your inability to concentrate, and thus you run from the situation and return to the drugs. Why? Because it is easier to avoid the reality that your life is slowly slipping away from your control than it is to actually take control. Eventually, your behaviors change so much that the people most important to you become concerned, but you claim there is nothing wrong. Sure, there is nothing wrong. It is a road that too many people have been down, and one from which it is difficult to return.

Alcohol in and of itself has its own effects, primarily on your liver and your heart.[33] Again, all the fun ends if you drink too much. Excessive drinking could lead to blackouts, vomiting, or even some extremes of choking on your own vomit while you sleep, which can lead to death.[33] Moreover, if you drink enough over the course of the evening without even realizing it, you may need your stomach pumped. Lastly, if you are so concerned with maintaining a certain body image and seek to create that all around balance in your life, drinking alcohol will only increase the weight in your stomach. You can also very easily develop that belly you have been trying to avoid. Alcohol is very high in calories.[33] Therefore, pay attention as to why you are choosing to partake in the act of drinking.

Cigarette smoking becomes addictive and expensive. The risk factors include heart failure, heart attack, lung cancer and other lung diseases, and other potential cancers.[33] Aside from the physical and psychological effects it has on the smoker (e.g., nervousness, relaxation), it also affects the health of those who surround you. Is that dirty, habit-forming rolled paper cylinder really worth standing outside in the rain and snow only to add toxins to your body? There is a reason smoking is no longer permitted inside ...many prefer not to have nicotine as a side dish with their entrées. The need for social acceptance is in part what drives adolescents (which includes folks in their twenties) to participate in these behaviors.[26]

If you enjoy doing what you do without any of these substances, you will never become reliant. Therefore, it may not be important for you to buy into the substance abuse square on your board game of life. Conversely, you may want to buy into making time to educate others on the negative impact substance abuse can have on your social and emotional world. If you are happy enough as it is with the way your life is going, then keep on that track. If you are fortunate to have your health without any complications that often emerge from chronic illness, why run the risk of damaging your health if there is no need to? Either way, you are given the choice if you roll the dice and land on that square at various points in your life. What you choose to do with that choice is up to you and no one else.

If there is something about your social life that is lacking, maybe in numbers, maybe in strength, maybe in activity, look into all your options before choosing the route of substance use and abuse. We all have a choice regarding what we indulge in. However, if you choose to pack your lungs, short-term memory, stress, and fears into a bowl and smoke it, what makes you think the fears you have will disappear? The smoke is only the beginning of a fire that will continue to burn unless you understand why you are making these damaging choices. So, as you come around your game board of life, pay close attention to the choices you are making when you land on the substance abuse square and affiliated social behavior.

Quick Points

- A drug high is only temporary.
- Smoking will not help you as much as you may think — pay attention to the effects.
- Understand that you have a choice with each interaction you have and the behaviors that come with it.
- Pay attention to what would make someone choose to use a substance.
- Where there is smoke ...there is a fire created that may be bigger than you will realize.

Notes Page
Thoughts? Feelings? Intentions? Actions?

_____

_____

_____

_____

_____

_____

_____

_____

_____

_____

_____

_____

_____

_____

_____

_____

_____

_____

_____

_____

_____

_____

CHAPTER 10
The Twenties and Far Beyond...
Mentally and Chronologically

"To get up each morning with the resolve to be happy...is to set your own conditions to the events of each day. To do this is to condition circumstances instead of being conditioned by them."
~Ralph Waldo Trine

As you approach various stages in your twenties, you ask yourself those same questions that you asked entering junior high and high school. The questions include: "Who do I want to be for the next four years?" "How will I define personal success?" "Who do I want to affiliate myself with?" "What type of person am I looking for as a significant other?" The same questions will continue to resurface in your life, but most likely the answers will be different. At this stage in your life it is less about what movie you are going to see on the weekend or which friends you choose to be offended by. The concerns become far greater as you start to move out on your own, making decisions that will eventually establish your life. Prior to your twenties, you were making choices that would help define who you wanted to be for the weekend or the year.

Now, in your twenties, you are making choices that will help define who you do and do not want to be for more of a long-term basis. You still have the big three to deal with: building your confidence, seeking a companion, and your response when surrounded by substance use and abuse. Yes, even well into your twenties and thirties the substance abuse issue will be present. Regardless of what happened in high school and college, the deeper you delve into your twenties and thirties you are given another chance to redefine yourself. You will be presented with choices that could better your self-esteem[27], raise your self-confidence[32] level, and enable you to gain optimal enjoyment out of life.

The difference between your teens and your twenties is that there are different issues you have to deal with. I am sure you have heard before that when you enter college you can make your own choices, choose your own career path, and be yourself. It is true that you pave your own path; the courses that go beyond mandatory material help to define who you are, what interests you most, and how deeply you want to study it. Your choices are no longer based on those of your friends. Beyond school, you pick and choose the activities and organizations with which you want to be affiliated. Doing so will give you the option to explore a variety of alternative fields, establish new friends, and enhance friendships that share these interests.

The key is to make a sincere effort to really get to know yourself. If you are most interested in business, give that a try. If you want to know more about law, psychology, poetry, art, or music, then that is your interest to pursue. Moreover, you can try all of these things until you find exactly what it is that most interests you. What you choose to do in your early twenties may vary greatly from your ultimate choice in your late twenties to early thirties.

As I was writing this chapter, I had a conversation with someone at a local restaurant. For anonymity purposes, it was decided her pseudonym would be "Ms. Iowa." I told her, "You have this time during your twenties to take chances before you settle on one path. Take advantage of this time you are given. Allow yourself to fail and embrace the success and confidence that comes along with it. Know that there will be different challenges throughout the process, and that is okay. It is most important that you always make time to stay true to your youth and your personal interests regardless of your age."

Building your confidence involves establishing yourself in areas that are most interesting to you, that help you better understand yourself, and will boost your morale and self-esteem.[27, 32] You may not be happy with all your choices. Much like other times in life, you will take some wins and losses. The bottom line is that you are still out there in the game and doing what you can to realize who you are. Another major aspect of the twenties, thirties, and beyond is how vastly different your social circle becomes. You start to make choices as to specific people you want to spend the most time with who may live in different cities. It is funny because you spend the first twenty years of your life attempting to build all these strong connections and fit into the "right group," wearing the clothes that will make you noticeable, or part of the mainstream trend. The difference with your twenties is you do and wear whatever you want.

Regardless of the chances you take, people might make negative comments or people might pay you compliments, but you will never know what is definitively you unless you try. You are beyond the nonsense that goes on in high school, so do it: be yourself; make your own choices when it comes to clothes, music, friends — and most importantly, significant others.

As your social circle decreases, the age range within your social circle increases as the gap decreases. So, someone who is twenty-seven can very easily find compatibility with someone who is twenty-one. But someone who is twenty-one may not so easily be able to relate to someone who is fourteen! Regardless of your sexual orientation[28], certain people who may have either been "out of your league" or "off limits" due to legalities or a sibling affiliation are suddenly not only in your league, but are playing in the same division. This is evident once you start seeing certain people at social gatherings who in years past were too young to attend. Initially it may be weird, especially if you have siblings in those age brackets, but you can get over that. If you are attracted to someone and they are playing the same game, why not approach?

The truth is that many people do approach others as the dating world changes in your twenties and well into your thirties. It may seem weird that you all of a sudden become interested in someone who is your older sister's age or older brother's age, or someone who has lived down your street for years. The idea of dating in your twenties is solely about interests, compatibility, and expanding your field of vision while maintaining respect, integrity — and above all, legality.

Compatibility is essential because the depth of the relationship is far deeper than those in high school. High school relationships (as mentioned previously) tend to be typically fun, light, and sometimes sexually driven.[29] Relationships in your twenties take on a whole new meaning, because you could very well be with the person with which you may spend the rest of your life. You start to establish yourself in your chosen career path, as does your partner. You move from apartment to apartment and perhaps from city to city and you make major decisions, such as whether the person you are with will come with you.

You are faced with major decisions. For example, are you dating to date for the short-term or are you dating for the long-term? Ask yourself that very question when seeking a mate and you will soon see the significant difference between the two. Regardless of what your intentions are, you want someone who is compatible, consistent, trustworthy, honest, and open to the exchange of communication. Without those major components, you may be basing your relationship purely on sexual attraction. Those seeking a significant other to be an important part of their lives beyond initial compatibility should focus on three cornerstones of a substantial relationship: trust, honesty, and respect. The beauty is that all three are integrated, but each is individually based because without one, you lose the foundation.

Individuals in their twenties and early thirties are primarily seeking similar aspects in a relationship. There are individuals seeking partners who will provide the least amount of excess baggage. Then there are individuals seeking a partner who is willing to show some sign of commitment – and, of course, limited excess baggage. Whichever of the two aforementioned individuals you can most relate to, pay attention to your preference without sacrificing your ideals. It is essential to have friends outside of your romantic relationship.

If you want to continue hanging out with your friends all the time, you may not be ready for a committed relationship. When you are involved with someone, it is important to give this person more time than you do your friends. By no means should the relationship be an all-or-nothing deal. If you have a significant other, make sure to still see your friends. If you have a large group of friends, make sure to understand that the significant person in your life is a significant part. Therefore, you may do things that you do not enjoy too much like watching football, taking dance lessons, going to the theatre, going shopping, taking cooking classes or hikes in the mountains for the afternoon, but that is okay.

We all lead busy lives and we already do not have much time for each other. So, when you do have time, you want to do something together. It all starts here, because it is just setting you up for your children or if you do not have children, it will help sustain a connection with your partner throughout life. Do you think most people want to go see some fifty-minute cartoon movie that costs twelve dollars admission and thirty dollars in snacks at the show? No, but you do it because your children want to go and you want to be with them. Do you think someone who does not enjoy ballroom dancing or attending a football game has a desire to go? No, but they go if it is an interest to their partner and helps the partnership grow, because that is compromise, that is support, and not obsession with the other person.

So, take note now in your twenties and get used to wanting to spend time with your significant other, even if it is an activity that you do not want to do. Let go of what other people may say or think. You do it because the other person wants you to, you are in a relationship, and know the other would do the same for you. You are learning new things about each other; therefore you are not just doing it for the other person or because they want you to do it — you do it because you want to be part of their interests. Additionally, you want to find a partner who also shares their deepest interests with you, so that the two of you can bond deeply over the things that matter most. Experiencing similar interests and ideals with each other will also help reveal to your children that you are unified on many levels or if you do not have children, you are communicating to your partner, I want this relationship to continue growing in all areas. Regardless of your different interests, you remain connected on the foundation of your relationship. You have the option to remain, two independent people with one unified heart.

In your twenties and beyond, you get to that point where you cannot have your cake and eat it too. If you sign on for the relationship it may help to show the other person that you are interested in their interests and it is not enough to either listen or pretend to hear. That is the biggest difference about dating, relationships, and partners in your twenties. You no longer hang out in large groups. You cannot always include everyone in plans. You cannot make a hundred calls, and send text messages and e-mails or internet social networking postings trying to get everyone in on the weekend plans. That ends as your teens and early twenties do. You begin to allocate certain times for certain people.

Sure, there will be events where it seems like everyone you know is in the same room, but that usually happens once or twice a year. On a daily basis your plans are centered on your small circle of friends and the significant other you are involved with or are in the midst of pursuing. You move from the concept of superfluous to specific when it comes to social circles.

Your friends start to change as you gain a better understanding of who you are. You work toward your specific career and away from commonalities. The regular scene of going out may become boring and repetitive after so many years. You may become quite happy with one person as part of a life partnership, leading you into the mentality that this one person could very well be the one person with whom you want to spend the rest of your life.

So what can you do about it? Grow, learn, pay attention, and apply a dedicated effort. In time, you may realize what you do not want, which can help to articulate what you do want. It is essential to think about what is going to make you happiest, compromising certain things without having to sacrifice everything you stand for.

You may not have been the most outgoing individual in high school or in your early teens, maybe because of discomfort about the way you looked, maybe because of the way you felt about yourself, maybe because of your lack of confidence, or maybe it was because of who your friends were. Whatever the case was, do not let how you were define who you are. Understand that the past does not define who you are; it is just part of where you once were. Use the resources you have. Enjoy the time getting to know someone at a deeper level, and if something comes of it, great — if not carry on with your own proactive game plan.

In your twenties you will be moving constantly; understand that, and be prepared for continuous change and uncertainty. However, it should not limit the people you choose to spend time with, which can include the concept of long-distance relationships. The long-distance relationship can be a result of a close connection to someone who might live in a different city or even country, but with whom you want a personal relationship. In your teens there is less of an investment, and I would not suggest dating someone in a different city, simply because you are young and you will change a lot in between visits, way more than you realize.

However, being in your twenties and thirties is different. The hope is that you spend this time meeting new people and learning about yourself. If and/or when you do eventually connect with someone from a different area code, there is no harm in trying the long-distance deal. Be prepared for intriguing night-time conversations that could last hours and cover more than just what you did during the day, and planned or periodic visits. This is not a part-time role.

For long-distance relationships to work, your mind and spirit must be in a full-time, dedicated, loyal, and trusting relationship. The lack of physical presence is to be balanced with an even greater mental, emotional, and verbal presence. You cannot express yourself with your body, so you must find other ways to do so. Snail mail is highly underrated—be creative. A long-distance relationship, on many levels, must be stronger than a local one to survive.

Of course, part of the reason why it can work more now than in years past is because of the numerous methods of communication. You can go through your day connecting with someone in at least six different ways without even being present (e.g., phone, mail, e-mail, fax, text, internet chat rooms, or webcam), but remember it works only if you are willing to put a greater effort into it. The reality, however, is that life does not stop. Your work and school cannot be put aside to facilitate this relationship. Do not forget that over ninety percent of communication is said to be nonverbal.[8] You have to be able and willing to work with that as you enhance and maintain a connection.

Life has to go on, therefore, in order for the relationship to work long-distance (again, it can if you believe it) you have to get to the point where you can live your lives while visiting one another. For example, if you have work to do, you do not put it on hold when you are together; you work while being together. It would not be so normal if you visited your significant other for seven days and she had work and you did not. Then you flew halfway across the country to be a hired boyfriend; all the while you are missing five days of paid work and not making any money visiting. As a result, some form of resentment may transpire which will cause a rift in the relationship, and the reality of distance will surface.

Thus, if you do choose to go the long-distance route, be prepared to carry your current life in a suitcase. If for whatever reason you cannot do that, then the long distance may become too long and the relationship will be cut short. Long-distance can work, especially if you want it to. Again, you will make the choice if you want it to work. Ask yourself three questions: "Do you think about this person all the time, especially when you go out at night?" "Are you uninterested in others?" and "Would it bother you if this person started dating someone else?" If you answered yes to those three questions, then you should disregard the distance and try it. Do not be afraid of failing. Moreover, understand that relationships that do not work are not failures, but learning experiences.

In a significant relationship in your twenties, if you do choose to take that step and move in together, be *very* careful that both of you are on the same page as to how you want to see things progress. It is important to know why you are moving in together and make sure both people explicitly communicate their reasons. One thing to avoid is moving in together because of convenience or because it makes financial sense. Your relationship is not to be some form of financial transaction; instead, it is a connection between two individuals outside of finances.

The person you plan to live with is not a business proposition or a client that you are willing to invest in to save you money in the long run. Living together sets the stage for a whole new chapter in your life. Be prepared to live with someone even if they may not turn out to be your life partner. Furthermore, just because you are living together, that does not necessarily guarantee that you will be together forever. It is another test in the question of "forever"? It is nice and fun to play house and pretend, but be aware of the differences between playing life partners and actually being life partners. Be prepared for both outcomes: 1. living together for life partnership, and 2. living together for the experience.

Once you get to the crossroads of what step comes next, be aware of the distinctions between planning a wedding ceremony and planning a life partnership. One is an event and the other is way of living. You are to understand that it is not necessarily essential that you live together before you obtain some legalized document acknowledging your lifelong devotion to one another. The hope is that you spend so much time together, understand so much about one another, and spend so much time at one another's places that each of you knows how the other lives. You are so synchronized with one another's emotions that you do not just finish each other's sentences — you complete each other's thoughts before and/or as they happen.

Emotions within a relationship are what create and maintain the heartbeat. Adding in destiny is not only powerful, but more so, enhances the emotional bond that is calming, challenging, and really brings the connection to life. Ask yourself what more you will learn about the person living with you that you do not already know?

Finally, in your twenties and early thirties, if you are with the person who you want to spend the rest of your life with, be sure to communicate how you want to live your life. For example, communicate what kind of neighborhood you want to live in, what kind of schools you want to send your children to (if you choose to have children), and how you want to spend your money. These are all major questions that can make or break any relationship. The key is to be honest with yourself even if it means letting go of someone you love. In this phase of your life, being honest with yourself and your partner is the only option. Remember the importance of honesty with your head, heart, and mind.

The idea that you move in with someone to "try it" holds only some merit. The rest of the questions fall into the category of what you are questioning about the person that you are uncertain of and therefore have to live with them to see. Aside from your professional life in your twenties and the time spent sleeping, you have the remaining five to seven hours per day to fill the void with some form of social interaction. As time limits increase, you prefer to have that one go-to person who becomes a significant part of your life.

Another aspect to consider as you march through your twenties is that of the drug world you became so used to seeing as you marched through your teens. The scene is just as evident if not stronger through your twenties. Why do people still not understand the effects by the time high school or college finishes? As you take on various forms of employment and funds are made readily available, chances are you can spend the money on what you enjoy most. For some folks, spending that money is directed toward rolling, lighting, and smoking.

The biggest difference between a teen who frequently uses drugs and an adult who does the same is that the adult does not have to answer to anyone. They are officially in control of their own lives (or so they think), and thus need only answer to themselves. Teens often have the ability to blame others for their dependence, such as parents whose presence is non-existent, school not educating the teen on the effects of the substances, or peer pressure. While the fault is typically that of the child, without taking responsibility they lean toward having scapegoats. However, as an adult, there is no one at whom to point the finger other than yourself.

The final point I will emphasize is the importance of open, effective, and assertive communication.[5, 30] The art of communication is such that you can express your thoughts, feelings, interests, beliefs, and opinions.[5] Whatever form of communication you tend to prefer in your twenties is up to you; just make sure you use it.

Effective communication with friends, significant others, and family will only enhance your relationships.

Too often it is easier for people to not say anything if it goes against the grain or might offend someone. Do not be afraid to raise important issues that may be hurtful or that may be difficult to talk about. It is okay to be uncomfortable talking about certain issues; allow for that discomfort and know that you and any relationship will grow from the experience. Again, I ask you: When you say to the world that you are an honest person, how honest is your communication when speaking with others?

It is important to be aware of the boundaries you can cross with certain people. You do not constantly need to tell everyone what you are thinking, but if there is something bothering you, know who to share it with — and most importantly, know how to share it. The most effective form of communication is not in what you say, but in how you say it. I spoke of various forms of communication in the mental and emotional balance section. However, I want to stress again how important open communication is in every relationship you are in.

With various forms of communication available today, it is very easy to say what you are thinking. However, it is just as easy for it to come out wrong, and the person receiving the message may not interpret it as you intended. If you are angry, happy, sad, frustrated, or excited, for whatever reason, share that information with someone. If you have friends who can read nonverbal cues, then you are lucky. Most people cannot see feelings unless you express those feelings.

Do not be afraid to communicate exactly what you are thinking and feeling. It will open all lines of honesty, trust, and genuineness.

By opening these lines of communication, the person or people on the receiving end will know what offends you, what makes you happy, or what irritates you most. If you choose not to share the feelings, you are hurting only yourself. For example, if there is something bothering you about certain family members or a significant other, what would be the harm in their hearing it from you? They may get angry or they may defend themselves against your comments, and this in turn may stir up a big verbal argument. However, by not releasing your thoughts and feelings to someone you care about, you are only *shooting yourself in the foot*, because each time a similar situation comes up, your level of being uncomfortable or upset will only increase. If these people are in your family and you cannot even tell them your honest thoughts, then who can you tell? Thus, share the comments and feelings, but be sure to know it is not what you say, but how you say it!

So how do you communicate anger, frustration, resentment, happiness, joy, or excitement? There are a number of different ways to communicate how you are feeling. As discussed earlier, verbal[15], physical,[16] and written[17] expression can be effective in communicating thoughts and feelings. However, the techniques used in communicating are a more detailed process of how feelings can be articulated. The key is to understand the difference between aggressive[34], passive,[35] and assertive[26] communication.

Aggressive communication is when you decide to point fingers at the recipient and say things like "I don't like it when you do this," "I hate it when you don't do enough of that." Whatever the sentences are, the sender is pointing fingers, and the receiver may respond in a defensive manner.[34] What is the most common response to offense? Quite simply...defense.

The second way you can communicate your thoughts and feelings is passive communication.[35] Passive people tend to just accept the criticism and allow their frustrations to build up but are unable to communicate their true thoughts because often they are afraid of being hurt or hurting the other receiver(s)' feelings.[35] They back away, curl up, and just hope time will pass without ever finding out what the person is hurting from or happy about. Personality style and type often dictate your behavior and communication style. However, there are ways you can learn how to communicate that may be most effective.

What seems to be most effective is assertive communication.[30] Assertive communication is an opportunity to communicate how you feel. You do not point fingers at the receiver; nor do you step back and allow your feelings and thoughts to build. The assertive communicator shares their true feelings and impact it is having on their lives.[30] Therefore, you are to make a statement like "I feel like I am not being heard," or "I would like to feel more appreciated." Understand what your true feelings are and articulate them in a way that effectively expresses everything you are thinking, ensuring that it is not an attack, but more an understanding, and be specific to verbalize include what you need, to avoid having the other person guess. The best part of assertive communication is that people cannot dispute your feelings. Only you know your feelings, and no one can take that away from you. Of course, there are people who will dispute and dismiss feelings. One way to help identify that is by noticing the moments when you are communicating your feelings and needs and the other person does not appear to be understanding why you are sharing these feelings and how important it is that you feel heard. For example: "I know you are telling me, I should not feel that way about spending time with your family, but I do and I would really appreciate your support when I am uncomfortable with how they speak to me."

The *how* of communication is one of the most difficult tasks, because if you do not feel confident in the response or you are afraid of the response, often you will hold back. Therefore, to help yourself better communicate in work relationships, friendships, romantic relationships, and family relations, understand how you feel and begin your thoughts and words with "I feel ... " and see how far that gets you. This is where the other forms of communication tie in well.

If there are a number of concerns you have that a boss, significant other, or family member may be hurting you, write them down. Write down everything that seems to be hurting you, then actively switch the words on the paper to "I feel ... " and then take the step and verbalize those feelings. The crux of assertive communication is maintaining open dialogue and decreasing any negative feelings that may be plaguing a relationship. You are simply stating your feelings and interests that will ultimately make you happiest.

Good communication is imperative to a good relationship, especially romantic. When it comes to communication, you can really judge whether a person is listening. We hear with our ears and listen with every other part of our body: eyes, face, body movements, heart, and legs. It can be very easy for people to hear; their ears do not do anything. Moreover, if they do not have difficulty hearing, they just have to sit there and hear what you have to say. To listen is a step toward actually concentrating on what you are hearing.

You can tell someone is listening when they nod their head, their eyes are looking at yours, and they make gestures with their body affirming that they are more engaged in the conversation, as opposed to being slouched back in their seats or looking away from you. Pay attention to both verbal and nonverbal cues and you will easily distinguish between those who are hearing you and those who are listening to you. Thus, to create open communication it is important to actually be a part of the communication process at all times. Communication in significant relationships is not a part-time gig; it is full time, so be prepared for it and expect that in return. Never ever keep your partner guessing, always tell them what you need, how you feel, and what you want.

It does not matter how old you are and how long your relationship has been going on — share your thoughts and feelings. We all have initial walls of trust that we do not necessarily just open up and share, but eventually you have to give that up and be willing to be honest, open, and encouraging. The only way to do this is through open and honest communication. Without consistent communication, you may drift as a couple; you may feel there is more out there for you, and it may build up levels of frustration and resentment toward the other person before you realize it.

If you plan to be with someone for more than a week, you have to be willing to let them into your life. You can see a strong relationship between sharing your thoughts and strengthening a bond, all by means of open communication. It is one thing for you to just agree with your significant other, but if they hear only an echo, then the relationship is not honest; chances are they would date themselves.

Share your thoughts, share your feelings, and do not be afraid to put yourself out there on the line even if it contradicts what your partner may think. What if your opinion contradicts another's? You discuss, you debate, you learn, and you grow. Always be accepting of others' opinions, even if they counter yours – it will lead to a greater open-mindedness and a more attentive ear to diversity. This is especially important to nurture an open and honest relationship.

Share what you are thinking and feeling any chance you get. Ask yourself: What is the worst that can happen if you are honest? It is not what your feelings are; it is how you choose to express them. It is important that you consider how you are being heard. If it is not necessarily as you intended it to be perceived, it could lead to additional problems. This is especially important when you are not sharing your thoughts face to face (e.g., in an e-mail). The key is to get the point across; otherwise you engage in a frustrating dance, and although dancing will have some missteps, it is supposed to be a thing of beauty.

The same applies to your friends. There are many things you may keep to yourself in fear of hurting someone, and that is okay too. However, if you feel close enough with a certain friend, do not be afraid to be honest and open in how you communicate. You will be making friends throughout your life, and creating that honest and open communication can either strengthen or sever your connection. If the connection is severed, then perhaps your connection was not strong enough to accept differing opinions; perhaps your characters clash too much to relate to each other at this point in your lives. Not saying anything, makes for a false, dishonest, and frustrating friendship. But again, when sharing your thoughts, be compassionate and sensitive as to how it is being heard.

If your connection is strong, you should feel comfortable enough to tell that person what you are thinking. If not, what will you talk to them about ... other people? Interesting people will talk about interesting things like thoughts, feelings, and emotions, with respect to themselves and the world. Boring people may have nothing to talk about so they will talk about ... other people. Gossip is the result of a lack of creative thought. Honesty will lead to credibility. Therefore, using honesty, your thoughts, feelings, and behaviors will be communicated in a balanced manner. Additionally, those with whom you communicate will feel closer to you. Your connection will be strengthened, as will your respect for one another.

Be aware of the changes that happen to you and

that many of the struggles you are having will continue into your thirties. You may feel you have balance in many aspects of your life at this point, but remember happenstance, opportunity, and penalties can occur. Thus, as you progress through your twenties and into your thirties, the board game does not stop; you just have the chance to roll again and keep playing if you so choose. The reality is with people marrying later and careers starting even later, struggles will continue. Thus, attending to how you cope with struggle in your twenties — and what works and what does not work — will help dictate how you proceed into your thirties. It all stems from how you choose to balance your communication style, relationships and connections you choose to establish and maintain as you progress through your twenties.

Quick Points

For a balanced, honest, and strong relationship:

1. Be aware of your strengths and weaknesses to tackle the social world confidently. Make a list of them, and add strengths and delete weaknesses as you see fit.
2. Try as many social activities as possible and then focus on the few in which you find success and enjoy.
3. Reevaluate yourself to make sure what you are spending your time doing is worthwhile, satisfying, and facilitates growth by doing one thing

every day that makes you happy.

4. Raise your self-esteem. If it makes you feel good about yourself without having negative effects on your health, then give it your all.

5. Do not be afraid to take a risk, join a group or activity. You will meet new people and experience something different. Therefore understand that relationships/friendships may not find you, and that you may need to find them.

6. Understand the difference between dating to date and dating for a life partner. Make the distinction and communicate your intentions.

7. Friends may hurt you, offend you, or put you down. Do not be afraid to confront them and do not be so eager to cut them off if it happens on occasion. We all make mistakes. It can happen with friends too.

8. Establish relationships with mutual understanding and respect, using open-ended communication.

9. Significant others will become a large part of your life, but ensure they do not become your life. Balance your time between your significant other, friends, and family.

10. Maintain a clear image of your relationships and friendships. Make sure you are in them for the right reasons and not just because it is easy and comfortable.

11. If drug behavior is an aspect of your life, evaluate what is pointing you in that direction and face the issue directly instead of pretending it is not there.

12. Alcohol intake may happen, but moderation is essential. Pay attention and do not use it as a method to alter your character.
13. Smoking – it can be addictive; try to avoid it at all costs in the hope of a proactive approach. It is a momentary relaxant, but coughing, shortness of breath, and damaged lungs are not that re- laxing, nor is paying for your weekly requirement and your medical bills. Smoking might even double the cost of health insurance. Read the facts. Your body does not deserve the beating.
14. Accept the ramifications of both wins and losses. Pay attention to how you can be better prepared the next time. Take advantage of the losses as an opportunity to gain a better under- standing of the situation.
15. Balance your time effectively. Pay attention to those with whom you choose to spend your time and understand that it is important to have more than one social outlet.
16. Take responsibility for your choices.
17. You can never say the words "thank you" enough to anyone. Say it and show it often.
18. Embrace change within yourself and those you are closest to.
19. Ask for help from friends and loved ones in your twenties; it is okay to show a sign of weakness.
20. Your turn ...add another.

Notes Page
Thoughts? Feelings? Intentions? Actions?

_____

_____

_____

_____

_____

_____

_____

_____

_____

_____

_____

_____

_____

_____

_____

_____

_____

_____

_____

_____

_____

_____

_____

_____

CHAPTER 11
Academic and Professional Balance – Anticipation and Preparation for Success

"You've got to get up every morning with determination if you're going to go to bed with satisfaction."
~ George Horace Lorimer

So you can balance your physical life, your emotional life, and your social life. However, keep in mind you have to be doing something with at least eight hours of your day. Whether it is school, a job, or any other form of work, there is a large part of your day that is occupied with some form of work-related tasks that will occupy your time. Ensure that work or school life has its own time and does not interfere with the other aspects of your life. Moreover, it is also essential that the other aspects of your life do not interfere with your school time or work life.

The main difference between school life and work life is that you bring school home with you. However, the more competitive the world gets and the more handheld devices that emerge, work life is being merged with home life as well. People are now bringing their offices home with them and eating dinner with their phones instead of their families. There is rarely a period of time when you are completely away from the office. Therefore, as much as you might desire to get out of school so you no longer have to worry about homework, you might find that work also crosses the boundaries of your personal life. We have the capacity, and are sometimes expected, to work from anywhere, whether it be in the kitchen with the family, on vacation, or while at the movies with your children or friends.

There is always going to be some work to do; how you fit it in depends upon how you allocate efficient use of your time. We all have schedules to attend to, but you need to be aware of the schedules of people around you as well. How do you balance everything you can in work and/or school life without overwhelming yourself, becoming too stressed, or neglecting important people in your life? To establish a balanced work and/or school life is to understand the importance of valuing other people's time, as well as your own.

If there is one thing you should take from this book, it is to learn to be prepared for the unexpected and to know you have choice with respect to how you respond to the unanticipated. The concept of being prepared versus reactive is illustrated in a quote by

Wayne Gretzky: "I skate to where the puck is going, not to where it is." It is all about anticipation and being prepared by planning ahead, both in your mind and in your actions (see example on graduate school applications, *Appendix D*).

So *when* setbacks happen, you are equipped with the resources to be practical instead of reactive. For example, if you choose to take a semester off of school in college or post-graduate studies, that is okay. One semester over a lifetime is equivalent to less than one percent of your life. If you have to take a step back from academics, that is your choice. Know that it is okay, and know that it can provide you with much-needed reflection time. It may be a setback in the moment, but it is a setback that will direct you down your chosen path.

Remember, every time you roll the dice you can land on happenstance or opportunity that could alter the daily routine or plan. Those simple words and the notion of anticipation hold true in every aspect of life, especially when it comes to work. Whether your game is ice hockey, business, teaching, or studying, as long as you are prepared and thinking ahead — as opposed to reacting to what is thrown your way — you are less likely to be taken off guard. Therefore, take any given day, start from the end, and work your way backward to the beginning. Think about what needs to be accomplished before the day finishes and plan how this can be done. Write it down, draw it out, or keep a schedule, (see *Figure 11.1*).

It will be a long time before you are ready to master this task of time management without writing it down.

Figure out everything you want to accomplish in your day, including work tasks, school tasks, meetings, social engagements, and time with your family. Once you have a list of everything that needs to happen, put the items in their order of priority. Then list the items that you want to happen, and choose wisely. It is not all going to get done in one day, and it is okay if you have to push certain tasks to another day.

You have a certain number of pieces to work with. Work or school will run you from eight o'clock in the morning until six o'clock in the evening. Dinner will hopefully take place after your day; then you may have an evening leisure activity for ninety minutes with some peers. The key is to make every attempt to be home by nine-thirty or later so you can lie in bed and read or engage in conversation to help yourself relax. So, where does the exercise come in? Try from seven o'clock in the morning to seven forty-five if you exercise at home, or a little earlier if you have to leave the house. Alternatively, you can take an hour out of your day, perhaps your lunch hour, and go for that workout and then eat a quick lunch after you exercise.

Therefore, you have exercise from six forty-five in the morning to seven forty-five, then work or school, followed by dinner, nighttime activity, and then relaxation. As night falls, prepare for tomorrow: make your lunch, pick out your clothes, and ensure that when you wake up in the morning it is not a replica of a fire-drill as you run frantically around the house trying to gather everything together. Plan ahead and expect setbacks. Now you have aligned all the pieces together and you are ready for the day.

School life has its crazy time too, with exams, tests, and projects. Work life brings about the same tornado, when certain times at work are busier than others. It happens to all of us; it is just a matter of how we deal with the incoming storm. Anticipate the storm, be aware that it is forthcoming, and be prepared as it approaches.

First Work, Then Play

Make sure you complete your day's work and leave time to do something you enjoy. Regardless of your age, complete your day with a hobby such as sports, painting, reading, or playing a musical instrument. Following this give yourself at least twenty minutes to relax and think about your accomplishments of the day and your goals for tomorrow. To optimize both work and play, find out what time of day you function best, as that is when you want to try to do your most challenging work and then earn your play time.

Prioritize

Get into a schedule that will help you prioritize your obligations, your activities, your family, friends, and your well-being. If you are a high achiever who is always seeking more and is never content with the task to label it complete, you may not be taking care of yourself in the process. It is important that you learn to walk away from your work at the end of the day to provide for a balanced life. This ensures that your day is diverse and includes time for yourself. You can fit it all in as long as you think about "where the puck is going." The key, again, is to work backward, deciding what you want to get done by the end of the day and putting the pieces in place to think about how it will look.

Start with the things you cannot control, the tasks and events that cannot be switched (e.g., a birthday party, a dentist appointment, a football game, work schedule), then place the pieces that work best for you in the available time slots. Embrace a four-P system: Prioritization, Patience, and Preparation, leading to Prevention. Know you have a choice in every facet of your work and/or school life. It is what you do with that choice that may help determine your priorities.

Sleep!

Ensure you have allocated a certain time for everything so that you are able to get to sleep at a decent hour. If you do not get a proper amount of relaxation and sleep, your ability to function will decrease. Again: preparation and anticipation; know what you have to do long before you have to do it. It is also important to be aware of the importance of a mid-day nap if that helps you function best later. It is okay to procrastinate as long as you are intentional about it and it does not distract you completely from your intended tasks. So, if sleeping in or napping is a form of procrastination, embrace it *within moderation*.

Get to It!

If you can learn how to establish some form of routine earlier in life, you will gain that much more in the future. Try to wake up every morning and say "I will do it all!" and then go to bed at night and say "I did it; now let's see what I have in store for tomorrow." There is no need to stress, panic, or worry about a test, a presentation, or a business meeting, if you are prepared. If you are the person who is always late, set your clock ten minutes ahead. Additionally, the "do it now" concept extends to making choices about your career, school, and professional development and exploring all your options along the way.

Part of the difficulty in balancing academic and/or professional stress emerges from making a choice as to what career path you want to follow. The process of going through the interviews is often enough for people to second-guess their career choices. For hints on how to master your school and/or job interviews, see Appendix E.

The reality is that your career path can and will change numerous times throughout your life, especially during your twenties. It is okay to try one degree path, realize you do not enjoy it, and then redirect your focus. Changing your career or academic path is not a failed attempt. The change is a barrier that is there to set you in the right direction and help you determine how motivated you are to seek and attain your goals. If you change as a person so much during your twenties, what makes you think your career path will not change with it? If part of balancing your professional or academic world requires you to spend time thinking about what it is you most want, then take that time at any point in your life, and know that is okay.

Regardless of what you choose to do with your professional or academic life, realize you have a choice, especially when you are open to it. Therefore, attend to your interests, but be mindful[14] of how you choose to spend your time with your work. Live in the moment and enjoy everything that is happening right before your eyes. However, be aware of what is coming (e.g., happenstance or unforeseen consequences at work or school), so that when it arrives you are ready for it.

For an example of how blocking out times during your week that you cannot control allows you to see the flexibility in your schedule that you can control, see Figure 11.1. The example pertains to a college student enrolled in a full course load of 12 credit hours. If you are not in college, adjust the schedule accordingly, starting with the obligations you cannot control. It may help you see that balancing your professional and/or academic life is possible.

It is your choice as to what you believe you want to be part of every day and items that you are only part of some days. In Figure 11.1, the black squares are parts of your day that you cannot or do not want to change, the gray areas are those that might vary from week to week, and the white squares are open times for you to fill in whatever you want. Look at the figure from afar and realize how much time you do actually have and make your choices accordingly.

Figure 11.1

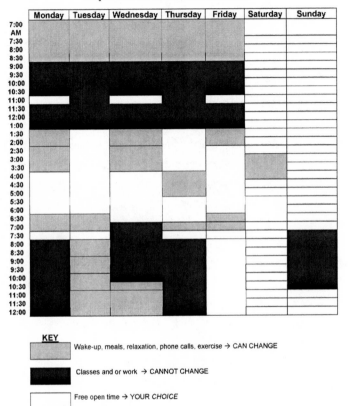

Daily Planner of Priorities and Preferences

KEY

Wake-up, meals, relaxation, phone calls, exercise → CAN CHANGE

Classes and or work → CANNOT CHANGE

Free open time → YOUR *CHOICE*

How do you do this? Here are some tips:

1. Have your clothes out and your lunch made the night before.
2. Write all your assignments in a to-do list and prioritize them.
3. Look at your planner or to-do list for the next day

and visualize how the tasks will be completed by working backward in your mind, allowing for set- backs.

4. Think about what you need to do by the end of the day and allow for each task to have a place taking you back to the beginning of the day. If you see that everything can be done in one day, this may enhance your motivation to accomplish it and do the same the next day.

5. Preparing and anticipating will allow for unforeseen circumstances to emerge and give you the power to respond effectively and not react impulsively or panic.

6. Do not forget a meal; if you do, it will make you less efficient and effective.

7. If you have homework, complete it before dinner while you still have energy, or at least an hour before you go to bed. You want to ensure you allow your mind and body time to rest before retiring for the night.

8. Allow yourself to take a time-out at least once during the day.

9. Be comfortable saying NO, sometimes. Not all of us wear blue tights and a red cape with a capital "S" on our shirts. Understand you cannot do it all.

10. Nothing is ever routine — allow for flexibility throughout your day.

11. Be sure to smile at least once during your day, if not more often. If you cannot smile, ask yourself why that is the case.

12. Concentrate on where you are choosing to

focus your energy to ensure it is being expended the way you want it to.

13. Share your feelings on the impact of your day with someone you love and someone who will listen.

14. Take twenty minutes before you go to bed to relax, enjoy your accomplishments of the day, wash your face, brush your teeth, and dare it be said ... even have time to floss.

15. Your turn again ... add another, and do not stop here.

There will be times in your life that are far busier than others. There will be times where your workload is far more demanding than normal. Just make sure the storm is only temporary and that there will be time for enjoyment. The last thing you want is for your family, friends, and leisure activities to become life obligations as opposed to lifetime enjoyment. Understand that life is not run on a military clock; you have flexibility, options, and spontaneity with your time as long as you allow for it.

Pay close attention to how easy it is for you to own these properties on your board game of life. Being a success may not solely be reflective of your bank account. Often times it is the simple spontaneous acts that invigorate and create excitement out of life.

Prepare for it, allow for it, and enjoy it – spontaneity is enlightening.

Does Spirituality Have a Place in Your Schedule?

Many people have an additional priority in their days and weeks: a religious or spiritual component. Having some form of connection to a greater being is important, as it can tie in well with a form of relaxation and fate. A religious connection may enable you to form a bond with something that extends beyond your own world. Some people find that a religious connection takes the mind away from work, school, your family, or your social life. I will not attempt to even begin to define religion or any spiritual connection, as it will look vastly different for everyone.

Some form of external connection may provide reassurance that your life makes sense — that all the stars are either aligned or are aligning properly, giving you an internal connection. Additionally, there is a purpose to your life; there is some pattern you are following, and this religious belief reassures you that you are doing okay. This greater being may also be there as a sounding board to help you process your thoughts. There is never going to be one right way of doing everything, and it is not possible to have everything work out exactly how it is planned. Therefore, you can dedicate a set time in your day or week to turn to a greater being to provide guidance and direction; however, it will look different for everyone.

Spiritual connection or religious affiliation spreads so far and wide. There is no one single generalized way to engage in religious activity or even begin to comment on how it can fit into your life. We are all different in some way, especially when it comes to a personal connection, multicultural differences, and preferences. For some it is simply important to feel that there is always some greater being watching over us.

Some religion can also provide for family traditions, annual celebrations, and reasons to unite. It can provide a social circle, acceptance, and an environment for discussion or debate. It may set values, fundamental beliefs, education, and a connection to the past. Everyone connects in a different way. You have to find what works best for you. You have to understand how much spiritual connection you seek, and where you choose to seek it. Upon understanding that, you then choose how much of a connection you wish to have and how important its presence is in your life.

Spirituality is a form of connection with another soul, another thought, another revelation. Whatever it may be for you, you must allow some form or capacity of spirituality in your life because it enables you to leave some life circumstances to chance and fate. As I recently discussed with my cousin Kylie, we all seem to live with a lot of uncertainty in life, regardless of the stage of life we are at. What will the future hold? Will my children be safe, healthy, and successful? How will I know that I chose the right career path, and when will that career start? Will I win the Little League championship? Will my friends now be my friends forever? The truth of the matter is, we cannot know too much about our own futures, as that may heavily influence how we live the present and prioritize our time. We have only so much control over what *will* happen, and thus all we can do is control how we respond to what *is* happening from one moment to the next.

There is never going to be a *right decision* when it comes to our personal or professional life, but there can be a choice that is our best fit for that time. Interests will change, friendships and partnerships will evolve, you will wonder "what if..." and the truth is that you have only so much time in any given day. It is not so much about the right answer as much as it is about some of the questions you might be too afraid to ask yourself. Take a moment to step back and ask yourself what is the worst that can happen, and then choose accordingly. Ambiguity need not be stressful, as it can be the one thing that maintains spontaneity in life, and that is what makes experiences so interesting. At the end of the day, you decide how you define happiness, success, and balance, which stem from each choice you make from one moment to the next.

Quick Points

- Plan your day backward, and realize it will all get done.
- Pay attention to what time of day you work best and use that to your advantage.
- Work hard, then play harder; value your free time, but be sure you are the one spending it.
- Schedule in time to delay the start of certain tasks. Not everything has to get done immediately. Spontaneous delays are permissible; just know you can procrastinate within moderation.
- Have faith, appreciate chance, embrace uncertainty, and believe in your potential.

Notes Page
Thoughts? Feelings? Intentions? Actions?

_____

_____

_____

_____

_____

_____

_____

_____

_____

_____

_____

_____

_____

_____

_____

_____

_____

_____

_____

_____

_____

_____

CHAPTER 12
Unnecessary Roughness: Embracing Chronic Illness

"Attitude is more important than facts. It is more important than the past, than education, than money, than circumstances, than failures, than success, than what other people think, say or do. It is more important than appearance, giftedness, or skill. It will make or break a business...a home...a friendship...an organization. The remarkable thing is, you have a choice everyday of what your attitude will be. We cannot change our past...we cannot change the action of others. We cannot change the inevitable. The only thing we can change is our attitude. Life is 10% of what happens to us and 90% of how we react to it."
~Charles R. Swindoll

As you continue to move through the spaces on your Monopoly® board of life, landing on the

Chance squares may not always lead to a positive outcome. Leaving some of life's circumstances to chance can be scary, especially with so much uncertainty in the future. You can intentionally make every attempt to balance each row of properties on your board game (e.g., professional, social, emotional, and physical) and still land on the receiving end of less-than-ideal circumstances. The reality is that a moment may change everything. The key to balancing the uncertain and less-than-ideal circumstances is to make every attempt to gain meaning and understanding of why and when this moment may have occurred in your life. A single moment can mean passing or failing an important exam, learning of a new pregnancy, receiving an incurable medical diagnosis, a wedding day, the day after your official retirement, a job promotion, a car accident, moving to a different city, or returning to your home city. Regardless of what the moment is that occurs in your life, the most powerful component can be recognizing what to do when that event happens, and how to process the effects and affect.

When questioned why I choose to make every attempt to live a life with intention, maximizing my health and experiences, I often respond: "Life can change in a moment, and I want to ensure I have nothing unresolved and no regrets." Living with no regrets takes risk; leaving nothing unresolved takes intention; and being mindful of each of your choices takes effort.

When life-changing moments happen, you will know how to respond. Whether these moments are life-ending or life-changing, your response to the situation is going to help dictate how you function thereafter.

Chronic diseases can happen to anyone. For example, you can eat healthy, exercise regularly, maintain strong ties with your family members, and work hard by giving back to your community and still be dealt a *2 of clubs* in your cards of life. I am sure you might be thinking: "If I make all the healthy choices in life and still get hit with the unnecessary roughness of developing a chronic illness or chronic disease, what is the point?" The same may hold true for your child or a family member, and you begin to wonder: "Why did that have to happen to my son or daughter [or my niece or nephew or my best friend]?" I will tell you this firsthand, because it happened to me.

After leading a balanced healthy lifestyle for over thirty years, one evening while I was driving, a car cut it front of me, leading to an unavoidable crash that eventually led me to the Emergency Room. Aside from the seven different injuries, I was diagnosed with Type I Diabetes. There are many lessons to take from these events that may help you better understand, accept, and embrace the less-than-ideal circumstances.

Unfortunately, chronic illness does not have any age restrictions. Illnesses that are more common in an elderly population happen to children and young adults. Illnesses that are usually diagnosed in children can unquestionably emerge later in life. Therefore, learning of a chronic illness can happen at any time and to anyone in life. Regardless of who it may be in your life that was diagnosed with some form of chronic illness (e.g., a parent, a sibling, a grandparent, a best friend, or even yourself), it is important to allow yourself time to first stop, step back, and sit with the reality of the diagnosis.

Even though the illness may not be instantly terminal, a recent diagnosis still requires one to grieve the life they once had, as if it will always be part of one's life. If it is you, your first thoughts might be mentally and physically rejecting the diagnosis, not believing you have it or not thinking that life needs to be that different once you leave the doctor's office. The truth is that many chronic illnesses are not life-ending, yet they are life-changing. Maybe not initially, but eventually, to maintain balance in your life, regardless of what the diagnosis is, embracing the illness will be important.

There are many chronic illnesses that may have impacted you and/or your family, such as: arthritis, cancer, chronic pain, Crohn's, diabetes, lupus, or stroke. Irrespective of the diagnosis or often multiple diagnoses, there may be a wave of emotions that can be overwhelming, and that is okay. There is no need to fight off these emotions to hide the hurt, the fear, and the sadness. If you are upset about the unfortunate information, be upset, be sad — and yes, it is okay to cry (men included). You may also feel annoyed, frustrated, nervous, and above all angry. Your emotions are all valid, as no one can tell you "you cannot feel that way." If you are angry at the situation or event, then be angry, because you have a right to feel the way you do. Just be sure these emotions do not consume your life.

Embracing the uncertainty of chronic illness will be an emotional experience; allow for it to be emotional, just not controlling. After all, you are learning a new phase of life and ultimately a new way to live life; it would only make sense for you to have an array of emotions, and that is okay. Your anger and sadness may lead to depressive symptoms. Your uncertainty, nervousness, and worry about the unknown may lead to or enhance anxious symptoms. These changes in your mood are all part of the process in understanding your circumstances.

After overcoming what might be initial shock when first learning about the change in health, you may be asking yourself: "Why? How? Where is the fairness in this world? What could I have done differently? Am I really a patient with this illness?" Although these are all valid questions and concerns, they do not change the reality of chance. Allow for those questions to emerge and remain present in the moment to help you welcome the affiliated emotions, communicate them, and progress — because you may never know the answer to many of those questions.

Even though you may want to show your strength in front of your children, siblings, family, friends, and coworkers, the longer you hold on to those emotions, the more likely they are to come out sideways. By sideways, I mean you may express an emotion that is unrelated to an event. It may appear to be a weakness for you to show emotion. However, I have often found those that are willing to be honest, open, vulnerable, and authentic with their struggles exemplify courage, confidence, and heart.

Upon processing and expressing the emotions affiliated with your diagnosis, the next part of balancing the life-changing event is to understand how you will work *with* it. You still have choices to make, and one of the most important is how you will go about living with the illness rather than opposing its impact on your life. Of course there will be better days than others and sometimes you might wake up in the morning and say: "I am having a bad day, I need to take this one off, and I will try again tomorrow." You are living with a lot of uncertainty as to how the illness will affect you on a given day, so allowing yourself to take a day for yourself to rejuvenate is not only okay, it is healthy. Although you may feel like you are walking around with Kryptonite, you do not need to be flying around your city with a flashy red cape. You are human, and you can do only so much with the circumstances you have been given.

On any given day it will be important to evaluate how much energy you can afford to use for various activities and tasks. If that means you cannot exercise, then use that time to relax; or there may be other days when you have to modify the amount of work you are able to accomplish; that is okay. If you have to decline social events to take care of yourself, that is okay. These circumstances that emerge on a daily basis are part of the process. They may not be pleasant, but they are part of the process nonetheless.

An important part of the process of working through embracing and balancing chronic illness is that as you better understand your circumstances, you must learn to recognize when certain responses become less helpful. Isolating yourself from social outings, repressing your emotions, and allowing for frequent thoughts of hopelessness can become unhealthy. If you find yourself engaging in the aforementioned behaviors and thoughts to such a degree that they interfere with life for many weeks and months, depressive symptoms can become evident. If you start to feel as if your energy is rapidly declining and there are no recognizable physical symptoms present, consider the mental health impact the diagnosis could have on your life. Moreover, understand that the mental health impact can be part of the healing process in eventually accepting your new reality.

Regardless of how many days, weeks, or even months it takes you to process and learn how to work with your chronic illness, realize that throughout it all, you need to be your own advocate and take the time to heal. Your physicians, specialists, psychologists, family, friends, and other healthcare professionals clearly want to help you, but they see a lot of people in one day and may focus on just one dimension of what you need. To help maintain the balance and reassurance in your life, ask questions, ask for resources, and explain in detail the struggles you may be having, because everyone experiences chronic illness differently. You are a person and not a list of symptoms. Allow for the people that you are working with to understand you and the impact the diagnosis has on you. If they are not proving to be helpful, you have the ability and the right to find someone else who can be. You are the one living with the chronic illness, and if you or your loved ones do not advocate for you, who will?

Learning how much control you have over what you can do may make it easier to accept your own reality and, even though it is different from others', it does not have to be worse. There is no clear explanation as to why this may have happened to you, and part of understanding your illness is accepting that reality.

There is no explanation as to why certain people are flagged with unnecessary roughness at different points in their lives. Mentally you can try to make sense of it by knowing you can use this as motivation for others to learn from your strength. Spiritually or religiously you can say things like: "God uses these moments as a way of reminding us to slow down, not take life for granted, and teach us lessons that we would not have had the opportunity to learn." Or "God would not have let this happen if She or He did not feel you could handle this."

Socially you may see this as a moment to realize who the important people are in your life and how much of role you want some to play, while you might not want others to be involved at all. Regardless of what angle you use to spin the scenario, there is no right way to even begin to understand why unnecessary roughness occurs in our lives or those of our loved ones. What you can begin to do is understand your circumstances, how you will work with them, and what type of support you want from those around you.

Outside of the professionals who attend to your physical and sometimes mental needs according to their job descriptions, there are the people in your inner circles who often reach out to support you. It is most common for every person in your world to ask what they can do to help. You may hear questions like: "What can I get you?" "What can I do for you?" "What do you need me to do?" In North America, we live in a *doing* society and therefore the natural reaction when an unpredictable event occurs is to do something or to fix something. Of course this can be helpful to an extent, but what is often missed is the idea of being present with another person rather than doing anything.

The idea of being present with someone is often ignored. Learning of any new diagnosis can be scary, dark, and lonely. Sometimes all a person might want or need is for you to be there with them in their moments of despair. Take a step back from doing and just sit with the person in the dark uncertain place without offering them any remedies except for your presence. We meet so many people in our lives, and yet we focus so much on the next steps that we easily forget the purity of each other and what a hand to hold and a heart to understand truly means.

Additionally, learning of a new diagnosis, or modifying how you choose to live with a diagnosis, will give you a moment to reflect on who the important people are in your life and why. We often wait until less-than-ideal circumstances (e.g., illness or funerals) to reflect on and express what type of influence people have had on our lives and how fortunate we are to have them help color our world. Do not wait for these moments — tell them now.

Sure, when you learn of a new diagnosis and how you will cope with it, chances are you will not be yourself and you will do things that are different from what you normally do. Understanding that certain friends who you thought would be supportive may not be — and conversely, friends whom you have not heard from in a while may be some of the most supportive people. If the people you want in your life are significant, it will be important to explain to them what type of impact the illness is having on you, and also to understand how it is affecting them. You may think they are not being supportive when in fact they either 1) do not truly understand your struggles, or 2) are scared when they see you go through so much and may be uncertain as to how to respond.

If it is someone else, rather than wondering what you can do, it may help to shift your focus to how you could be of help and asking the person directly what would be most helpful for them. It may also help if the friend clearly specifically expresses what they are able to do and what they are good at. For example, I am available on Saturdays if you want me to get your groceries, take care of your children, or help clean your house. Experiencing, chronic illness is hard for everyone involved and being actively present rather than providing generalizable words of supposed comfort is important. Trust me, I am certain they do not need any reminders that dealing with their illness "must be tough" — they are pretty aware of that. Sometimes all it takes is your presence to shift the focus from the illness to the person. It will be important to talk with them about life outside of the illness, taking a vacation from the diagnosis and discussing their interests and their passions. Engage in discussions about the most recent award show, the last movie they watched, or who they think will win the Super Bowl.

It is not so much about what you can do to make them feel better — or sadly, what some try and do to make themselves feel better — it is about being present with the whole person, providing them with options, often validating their experiences, their lives, and their moments. Of course, depending on the illness, they may want to focus the conversation on the end of life, on their life highlights (e.g., school science fair success, Little League championships, past relationships, or favorite summer camp moments). As difficult as it may be to reflect with them, knowing time may be limited and the interactions and memories will look different, remember this is not about you, it is about how you could be of most help to the person with the diagnosis.

Regardless of your knowledge of the illness, you have not "walked in their shoes" to know how the diagnosis is truly affecting them. Every person is affected differently by a chronic illness. Try your best not to project what you think they are going through; rather give them the safe, comfortable, and supportive space to share their experience with you.

Both the individual with the diagnosis and the supportive people in their world who embrace the reality of the chronic illness will consistently wonder why bad things might happen to good people. I have been fortunate to share with my students and have talked about this many times over, wondering why bad things often happen to good people. One explanation is that most people may not really listen as attentively to *bad* people, yet they often have their ear to the floor when *good* people speak. Of course that does not change the reality of the diagnosis, but perhaps can shed some light on how you can use this experience to be an active instrument of change in this world that you may not have otherwise embraced. Regardless of age, we all have the power to be mentors; learning from one another, teaching one another, and inspiring people to pay it forward.

It does not matter so much whether the chronic illness is mental or physical; there are many people in your everyday life who live with invisible illnesses that are either masked by other activities, ignored because of how consumed we tend to be in our own lives, or just less obvious because they are difficult to see from the outside. It becomes quite impressive what some people are capable of when experiencing so many struggles in their lives.

As you continue to roll the dice on your Monopoly® board of life, recognize that chronic illness can happen at any given moment. Leading a healthy lifestyle prior to a diagnosis may not have prevented it, but it will help you adapt to it, and will also help with the lifestyle change.

Therefore, as you continue to create your path in life, each time you roll the dice, take risks and create adventures, travel, and learn about this world and yourself with each moment. Recognize how lucky you are to have the health you do. If you have 100 points of energy in any given day, ask yourself how many you want to devote to seemingly smaller stressors that can be resolved by changing your perspective. It is very easy to take advantage of life before a doctor tells you that you need to make drastic changes. Why wait?

Just remember that life will return to normalcy, even if that means you have a new normal. Even with what may feel like a set of broken wings, you will fly again regardless of how long it takes. The distance and destination of your journey may look different, and that is okay. You will experience moments in life that will unfold because of how you choose to respond to your circumstances. Sure, you may say things like "It's unfair," because it is — and you will be okay whatever that may look like. Stop, step back, and look around you. Look at the inspiration, courage, resistance, and perseverance of so many who have been diagnosed with any form of chronic illness. Remain patient, mindful, and never ever give up!

Even though at times you may feel like you are running into the wind, fighting a battle with cardboard, your feet stuck in concrete while wearing Kryptonite around your neck, you can enjoy your moments. You cannot change your circumstances, but you can change your attitude. You are still the axis to your world; you control the speed and direction in which it turns, and how each moment is defined.

Quick Points

- It is okay to express, show, and communicate emotion, especially when diagnosed with a chronic illness.
- Although there may be similar diagnoses, everyone responds differently. Respond to your chronic illness your way, especially maintaining a realistic attitude.
- Be your own advocate. Ensure you are getting what you need medically, psychologically, emotionally, and socially.
- When supporting a loved one or friend with an

illness, focus on being present with them rather than trying to do something or fix something.

- Try not to take your health for granted, as life can change in a moment — and if it does change, never give up!

Notes Page
Thoughts? Feelings? Intentions? Actions?

_____

_____

_____

_____

_____

_____

_____

_____

_____

_____

_____

_____

_____

_____

_____

_____

_____

_____

_____

_____

_____

_____

CHAPTER 13
Making the Impossible...Possible

"Don't wait until everything is just right. It will never be perfect. There will always be challenges, obstacles and less than perfect conditions. So what. Get started now. With each step you take, you will grow stronger and stronger, more and more skilled, more and more self-confident and more and more successful."
~Mark Victor Hansen

You may believe it is impossible to act on all of the suggested tactics in this book. You have to begin to train your brain to say "I can do this and I can do that, so as long as I take the more proactive, positive, and realistic perspective." Sure, you may fail at times, and at others you may succeed — but the key is to make every attempt to understand that you *can*. Replace all of your *if, and,* or *but* statements with *I want to, I will,* and *I can*. Set aside time to figure out what you want, how much of it you want, how you will go about getting it, and if you cannot attain it, what is the healthy alternative? The concept of life can be narrowed down to a five-category method that I call *THE PC* method.

We are all faced with difficult challenges in all four aspects of life: social, physical, mental/emotional, and professional. Each of us has our own quirks, issues, concerns, and stressors. Someone living in the exact same situation may have similar concerns, but no two people are alike in terms of what is holding them back.

Therefore, you have to take what is going on in your life as an individual and original situation; do not relate it to another person's experience. Related to this, you cannot achieve a goal by following someone else's path. The turns, crossroads, and forks toward reaching your goal are as individualized as your fingerprints.

Thus, I will conclude by helping you reframe your thought process as you move through the four quadrants of life. The hope is that you will attain your desired level of balance each and every time you roll the dice to play your board game of life. You will focus your energy less on trying to knock down others' houses and hotels, and more on building your own success. Concentrate on using your available resources and pay attention to *THE PC* model of thinking, feeling, and acting.

T.H.E. P.C.

T – Timing

Many things in life are about timing. These are things we cannot control, nor should we try to. However, it is important to maintain a proactive approach to life, all the while understanding that timing has the power to work against us. This is important, for instance, when sitting in traffic; it is understandable that you get frustrated. We all have important places to be, things to do, and traffic can impede that. The healthiest way to respond to it is to take a deep breath. Understand that traffic (or anything like it) is one of those realities that we cannot control, but we can control how we react to it. It may be bad timing that we caught a train while rushing to another meeting, but it happens. What is in control is your response.

As another example, many begin to grow impatient waiting for that great job opportunity, raise, or significant other to come along. Sometimes we can try our hardest and still be left empty-handed. Again, frustration can be kept at a minimum and hope can be maintained. Sometimes the simplicity of being in the right place at the right time plays enough of a role to reward us in the search for our desires. Thus, realize that even though your goals may be within reach, it may not be the right time. However, your proactive role in this sense is to keep trying, keep applying, keep interviewing, keep dating, and eventually timing will factor in on your side.

I quote the legendary Dr. Martin Luther King Jr., who when referring to faith, said: "You don't have to see the whole staircase, just take the first step." Sometimes timing works in your favor; sometimes it works against you. However, just be aware that your life story will unfold. Patience and a maintained proactive approach can be keys to succeeding. Do not give up — maintain your resilience, and keep trying.

H – Honesty

It is essential to be honest in everything you do. Every time you are dishonest with someone or even with yourself, take a step back and ask yourself what it is that drives you to stretch the truth or simply lie. Being true to yourself and to anyone with whom you interact will create a sense of consistency for you — honor, credibility, and value for your own self-worth and others who seek loyalty.

Honesty spreads from your home life with your family, to your friends at school or work, to your teachers, bosses, and everyday people. By being honest you have nothing to hide. By being dishonest, you are creating more work for yourself, as you will have to attempt to recall whom you told what, without missing a step. Again ask yourself: What would be the purpose of not telling someone the truth?

There are circumstances in which one may need to refrain from the truth. For example, protecting someone from something you believe would be a lot worse if they heard the truth. If you do know information that may hurt or impinge on someone's overall well-being or progress in life, you do not necessarily need to lie. However, sometimes you can remain honest by simply not saying anything. However, I would also ask yourself what is preventing you from disclosing something about yourself to the people most important to you. Be sure to distinguish between lying and avoidance.

If you think you should lie, ask yourself whether or not you need to say anything at all. Just because you know something about someone does not mean you have to share it. This indiscriminate sharing is gossip, and no one wants to be known as a gossip. You will hear time and time again that honesty is the best policy, and in most cases that is true. Dishonesty, as I have said many times, forces you to backpedal your way into a deeper rut. In the end, you will hurt more than you will help. Be honest, open, and up front, especially when it comes to friendships and relationships with everyone in your life. However know what is meant by private information and know what information may damage someone's feelings, health, or safety.

E – Effort

I cannot stress this enough—the things you want will not arrive at your doorstep or be fed to you with a silver spoon. You have to be prepared to put a serious degree of effort into everything you do. We are all given different materials when we are born, and it is up to you to make your story a success, by your definition.

When you do have to get down to business and get that assignment done, show your kids you love them, pay attention to your whole family while not neglecting your friends, maintain a long-lasting healthy relationship with a significant other, or compete in athletics, art, or music, it will require effort in pursuit of your desires. No one is going to do it for you. To reach your desired level of success, be prepared to put in the effort to earn your rewards, taking responsibility for your actions without cutting corners.

It is not what you do, it is how you do it that will effect your motivation to continue. Do not be afraid to grasp the idea that just because "it" is hard, that does not necessarily mean it is unattainable. Remember, if it were easy, everyone would do it. With difficulty comes challenge, and with challenge comes effort. If you love something or have a desire for something so much that you will put forth any degree of effort to attain that realistic goal, do not tell me you cannot so you will not — start thinking and saying that you can, and therefore you will.

P- Patience

I have touched on a lot of life aspects, goals, behaviors, and thinking patterns. The reality is that these changes cannot and will not happen overnight. As long as you are taking healthy steps toward your goals, with clear, realistic and logical thinking, feeling, and action, your desires can come to fruition. School decisions may not be certain for another two years; your career may be undecided for another five months or five years (in this day and age ten years really); the next person you date, or your next social outing may be something unknown to you for a little while — but be patient; things will progress. Life is a process and it takes time to unfold. As your stress level increases, it will be very tempting to lash out at a parent or other family members, friends, your coworkers, or a teacher. However, recall they are not going through the same things you are, and they may not understand exactly what is happening in your life, nor are they likely responsible for it. Be patient and help them understand; explain why you may be on edge; career decisions and such alike will occur when they do. Trust the process.

One of the hardest things about going to bed each night is not knowing what is going to happen the next day, and consequently feeling all the pressure of uncertainty. Be patient and do not feel you need to rush anything and everything. If you are fifteen, then be fifteen and do not rush yourself to be eighteen or twenty-one. Chances are pretty high that you will get to twenty-one, thirty-one, and forty-one. So, be patient and do not rush the process. Do not force yourself to enjoy the moments that are forthcoming later in life; enjoy the moments that are right now and be patient for the others to come. Do not let age force you to make decisions. As my friend Sarah eloquently said when I was trying to come to terms with the process of aging, "Age is the cost of experiencing life."

Developing a greater ability for patience will help decrease your stress level and increase your general congeniality around others. Not everyone works, thinks, and acts like you. We are all human and we are all different. Be prepared to accept that, and be patient. Everyone has stress, so if things are not working like a well-oiled machine, be patient, be aware of it, and work to change it. If you cannot wait for a red light to turn green, then you have to step back for a few minutes and let yourself breathe. As the Chinese proverb goes: "One moment of patience may ward off great disaster. One moment of impatience may ruin a whole life."[36]

C- Control

Finally, the "C" word: control. As I have mentioned earlier, be aware of what is within your control and what is not. I will take it all the way back to the beginning, and remind you we all start with the dice in our hands and have only so much control over what happens once we roll. The focus of our control does not come from how the dice land. How we choose to handle the outcome once they do land on the board is what is in our control. We all know we cannot control everything, and thus cannot worry about things that are out of our hands. Much of our worry stems from uncertainty. All we can do is take control of what we can (e.g., the hours of studying, how often we eat, which schools we can apply to, who our friends are, how often we spend time with our family, or the type of work we are interested in doing throughout life).

The things that are out of our hands (e.g., which school you will be accepted to, if an accident prevents you from getting to your meeting on time, or if the conflict in the Middle East will ever end) are all but unknown. Worrying less about the things you cannot control will help you focus on what you can. Too often we wrap ourselves up in incidents, situations, or scenarios that we cannot control. We worry, we lose sleep, we lose appetites, and in doing so we lose a grasp on our main objective in life-balance. Look back at the goals you set for the week, for the month, or even for the year and make every attempt to focus on those goals over which you have some control.

"Time is the coin of your life. It is the only coin you have, and only you can determine how it will be spent. Be careful lest you let other people spend it for you."
~Carl Sandburg

We each have only so much time here, and we tend to spend a lot of it trying to get somewhere, or reach for something, but never stop to think. We often neglect to think to ourselves: "Am I really doing what I love, and if not, what would make it better?" "Am I putting the most amount of effort I want to into my family, friends, myself, and work — and if not, why?" Know that as you attempt to monopolize your life on your own board game, you will repeatedly pass the happy birthday square, may land on the good fortune square every so often, or seldom have to re-strategize in the consequence center.

Whatever the case may be, the dice will keep rolling as long as you continue to play. Be aware of each moment you have and what you choose to do once the dice are rolled. Each turn you take may seem slow, but if you take the time to reflect, you will see your board game of life moves quickly. Attend to the interests that maintain your youth and the things that will continuously make you happy and fulfilled (even if that means waking up early to watch cartoons).

We live in a fast-paced environment where the deeper we move into the technologically advanced world, the further we move away from person-to-person interaction, contact, and communication.

We become uncomfortable with social contact — so much so that we call numbers hoping to get voice-mail, while relying on credit-card-sized phones and wireless communication from practically any location.

We tend to focus our attention too much on where we are going, and not enough attention on where we are, and what or who we are fortunate enough to have in front of us. Feel the necessity to engage in and appreciate the process to understand and optimize a balanced outcome with the people you choose to meet — and above all, yourself. It is a long and winding road. No two people will ever live the same life. So, pay closest attention to the ride and the people you let into your life along the way. Be sure to say thank you every day — even if you think it is unnecessary or might be assumed, say it. Remember that each time you pick up the dice to roll, remind yourself: "This is my life and I will make my choices." If our lives are comprised of choices and effort put forth to ensure moments are enjoyed, how will you choose to spend yours? Therefore, I ask you:

"If I gave you a clean sheet, what would you write? Would your words be long and graceful or short and sweet? Would it be poetry, or just plain English? If you have something to say, say it now. For soon, and always too soon, my sheet will be filled and this chapter will end as soon as the next will begin; with a clean sheet, new authors and a million possibilities."
~ Bauer Hockey

Good luck out there, and be sure to enjoy your choices that help define your moment!

The Paradox of Our Age
By: Dr. Bob Moorehead[37]

The paradox of our time in history is that we have taller buildings but shorter tempers; wider freeways, but narrower viewpoints. We spend more, but have less; we buy more, but enjoy less. We have bigger houses and smaller families; more conveniences, but less time. We have more degrees but less sense; more knowledge, but less judgment; more experts, yet more problems; more medicine, but less wellness.

We drink too much, smoke too much, spend too recklessly, laugh too little, drive too fast, get too angry, stay up too late, get up too tired, read too little, watch TV too much, and pray too seldom. We have multiplied our possessions, but reduced our values. We talk too much, love too seldom, and hate too often.

We've learned how to make a living, but not a life. We've added years to life, not life to years. We've been all the way to the moon and back, but have trouble crossing the street to meet a new neighbor. We conquered outer space but not inner space. We've done larger things, but not better things.

We've cleaned up the air, but polluted the soul. We've conquered the atom, but not our prejudice. We write more, but learn less. We plan more, but accomplish less. We've learned to rush, but not to wait. We build more computers to hold more information, to produce more copies than ever, but we communicate less and less.

These are the times of fast foods and slow digestion; big men and small character; steep profits and shallow relationships. These are the days of two incomes but more divorce; fancier houses but broken homes. These are days of quick trips, disposable diapers, throwaway morality, one night stands, overweight bodies, and pills that do everything from cheer, to quiet, to kill. It is a time when there is much in the showroom window and nothing in the stockroom. A time when technology can bring this letter to you, and a time when you can choose either to share this insight, or to just hit delete.

Remember, spend some time with your loved ones, because they are not going to be around forever.

Remember to say a kind word to someone who looks up to you in awe, because that little person soon will grow up and leave your side.

Remember to give a warm hug to the one next to you, because that is the only treasure you can give with your heart and it doesn't cost a cent.

Remember to say "I love you" to your partner and your loved ones, but most of all mean it. A kiss and an embrace will mend hurt when it comes from deep inside of you.

Remember to hold hands and cherish the moment, for someday that person will not be there again.

Give time to love, give time to speak, and give time to

share the precious thoughts in your mind.

AND ALWAYS REMEMBER:
Life is not measured by the number of breaths we take,
but by the moments that take our breath away.

Notes Page
Thoughts? Feelings? Intentions? Actions?

_____

_____

_____

_____

_____

_____

_____

_____

_____

_____

_____

_____

_____

_____

_____

_____

_____

_____

_____

_____

APPENDIX A
Progressive Muscle Relaxation[2]

- Begin in a quiet place, free of any potential distractions.
- Either lie on the floor or sit comfortably in a chair.
- Begin to slowly close your eyes.
- Start to take a deep breath in, followed by a deep breath out.
- Once you feel you are ready to begin take a long deep breath in, hold it for five seconds and then slowly release a deep breath out for ten seconds.
- Repeat the breathing technique until you feel you are becoming more relaxed.
- Once you are ready for the body parts, progressive relaxation will begin. For each body part it is important to:

1. Hold the tightness for five to seven seconds; squeezing as tight as you can, almost making a muscle with that body part, experiencing the

true sensation of the tightness.

2. Slowly begin to release the pressure, allowing for your mind, heart, and body to feel the sensation of relaxation.
3. Release the pressure for 20-30 seconds.
4. Engage in steps 1-3 twice for each of the following body parts:

    a. Forehead
    b. Eyes
    c. Jaw
    d. Shoulders
    e. Left bicep
    f. Left forearm
    g. Right bicep
    h. Right forearm
    i. Chest
    j. Belly
    k. Left thigh
    l. Right thigh
    m. Left leg
    n. Right leg
    o. Left foot (including toes)
    p. Right foot (including toes)

- Once you have released the tension in all of the above parts, return to slow deep breathing, holding the breath in for five seconds, and then releasing it for ten seconds. Once you are ready, slowly open your eyes.
- Also note that you can include more parts of your body as you see fit. You can also eliminate

some of the parts mentioned above if you are choosing to shorten the exercise.

- Find a time of the day when this is most effective and needed.

* Adapted from Jacobson, E. (1938). Progressive Relaxation. Chicago: University of Chicago Press. For more information see citations affiliated with number 2 in the reference section at the end of the book.

APPENDIX B
Exercise Plan

The information below is a sample of an exercise plan. For more information as to what each of these exercises look like, consult with your local fitness center if you choose to engage in the regimen below. I would also suggest discussing your desire to engage in exercise with your doctor before beginning any routine. The display of the numbers for each exercise is as follows: the first number equals the sets, the second number equals the number of times you do the exercise per set. For example, "3 x 12"= three sets of twelve repetitions in each set. Lastly, this is a suggested plan and it will need to be modified based on ability and strength. Above all, be sure to stretch before and after each day of exercise.

ARMS:

1. 5 lb weights standing still & raise arms to eye level 3 x 12 (*shoulders*).

2. 15 lb weights standing still & do hammer curls 3 x 12 (*biceps*).

3. 15 lb weights sitting on the flat bench and place your elbow on the inside of your leg and curl the weights. No breaks; right arm, then left 3 x 12 (*biceps*).

4. Lying on the incline bench, take 20 lb weights and bring them over your eyes 3 x 12 (*chest & shoulders*).

5. Lying on flat bench with 20 lb weights, turn the weights so your knuckles will face each other & bring weights over your eyes while 3 x 12 (*chest*).

6. Bench press, keep your hands either shoulder width apart or right beside each other 3 x 12 (*chest & shoulders*).

7. 21s: holding a long bar out in front of you at ninety degrees and curl the bar up to your face. Complete 7 repetitions with your hands right beside each other, 7 repetitions with your hands shoulder width apart, and 7 repetitions with your hands spread apart and let the bar roll to your fingertips. If the bench press bar is too heavy, use a shorter straight bar (looks like the bench press bar, but it is shorter and not as heavy) 3 sets (*biceps, chest, forearms*).

8. Sitting at the preacher curl bench, with your

arms hanging over the padding, pull the small (curved) bar upwards while someone is resisting your force. Get someone to spot you and make sure you work for it. It is not the same exercise if you add more weight to each side, it is the resistance that makes the difference. Place 5 lb weights (or less to start or more as you progress) on each side (*biceps, shoulders, chest*).

9. Sitting at the incline bench take 10 lb weights and do the curls with palms facing up 10 x 20 (*biceps*).

10. Abs: Use the rope on the pulley system, (put the pin in at a level you are comfortable with) and do 3 sets of as many as you can. Also, in a separate exercise, take 5 lb dumbbells, hold them together, place them over your head and do a standard crunch, bringing the dumbbells forward as you move.

LEGS:

1. STRETCH!!! Using a foam roller to stretch your legs is usually best.

2. Abs exercises, especially with a balance ball.

3. Use the machine where you lie down on your stomach and curl your legs up.

4. Place the long bar over your shoulders, get into the squat position, but then keep your left knee bent and stable while you slide your right leg outward (similar to skating). Repeat this step with your right leg 10 times, then switch to your left leg 10 times. Add weight as your strength improves.

5. Squats: Put 20 lbs on each side and squat down to the point where your knees are at ninety degrees but making sure your knees do not come over your toes: 3 x 12.

6. Lunges: Hold 5 lb dumbbells in each hand and take one knee down in the lunge position, then the other knee. Try doing this as you walk around a track or in a stationary position for 5 minutes.

7. Lunges with a weight: Hold a 5 lb weight in your hands and place it in front of your face. Then lift the weight above your head as you bring your left foot forward and lower your right knee. Complete this motion 10 times with one leg and then switch.

8. Run, elliptical, bike, spin, or swim for approximately 35 minutes, which includes cool down for 2-3 minutes.

9. Push-ups: Put two small dumbbells 3 feet apart and place your hands on top of them and do 3 sets of as many as you can.

10. STRETCH!! I am not kidding. Unless you want to make eventual and frequent appearances at the physical therapist, be sure to stretch before and after ANY form of routine exercise. If you are uncertain as to which stretches would be best for you, be sure to consult with the appropriate fitness consultant or health professional.

APPENDIX C
Meal Plan

It is important to note that the menu items provided below can be modified as needed based on nourishment needs or allergies. Furthermore, the items are generally low in fat, salt, and sugar and are intended to provide optimal nutritional, psychological, and physiological benefits. If certain items are not on the list, find out why before you choose to add them to your diet. Additionally, the items below are intended to provide optimal effects for a well-balanced diet. The hope is that these items below or any combination of them may help decrease stress and digestion difficulties, and increase happiness, energy — and most importantly, your productivity.

Similar to everything else in life, all eating habits can be optimized in moderation. The meal plan below is merely a suggestion; alter it as you see fit, but be aware of why you are choosing to make the substitutions. The menu below is not a "diet," meaning it is not something that is intended to be temporary. The menu is intended to be a lifestyle change that may help balance your digestive system, your mind, and your body. Lastly, if you get into the habit of reading nutritional labels on the side or back of the products, pay attention to the serving sizes that they include. Although some of the numbers may vary, seeming like an item is low in fat or low in sodium, take a closer look at the measurements they are using.

Breakfast:
Oatmeal

Eggs

Kashi cereal

Special K Protein Plus

Fiber 1

Yogurt (e.g., Fage or Liberte), fruit and low-fat granola (be very careful of the sugar content, as many types of granola and yogurt have a lot of sugar).

If you want to diminish your bread intake, limit it in the morning, but have it at lunch if you prefer

~10:30 a.m. snack

Fruit that is high in fiber (e.g., blueberries, raspberries)

Yogurt

Vegetables, especially those that help decrease stress and aid in digestion within the gastrointestinal tract (e.g., red peppers, cauliflower, broccoli, spinach or carrots)

Mixed nuts (almonds, macadamia nuts, seeds, walnuts, and some raisins and they add in digestion)

* Not salted – that is often counterproductive! Mixed nuts that are salted have a tremendous amount of calories as they are heavily coated and can diminish the nutritional benefits. All nuts are high in calories, I suggest eating those that are unsalted or flavorless for optimal benefits (e.g., raw almonds).

Cheese (one serving size, 1 ounce or 28 grams though) and low-fat crackers

*Too much cheese can impact your cholesterol and caloric intake.

Lunch:

Sandwich – (turkey, veggie, chicken, salmon, hummus, cheese, tuna, steak – only whole-grain bread)

Salad — load it with ingredients that are all high in protein and/or fiber (e.g., raisins, fruit, almonds, chickpeas, eggs, tuna, cheese, broccoli, and avocado)

Vegetables (same as 10:30 a.m. snack above)

Chips or unsalted pretzels (not regular try and find the baked options as they may better for you, usually containing less oil).

Fruit as a side

*Note: careful of the dressing. You can get a salad anywhere that is loaded with goodness, but if you put a lot of Caesar dressing on it, for example, you are better off going with the Big Mac. Most salad dressings (especially creamy dressings) and salads that contain deep-fried meat at fast food restaurants have more calories than the sandwiches.

~3:00 p.m. snack

Similar to the morning snack options (note: protein bars are not an optimal snack, while they are high in protein, they are equally high in sugar. Thus, fat-free now... often leads to more fat later, meaning an increase in sugar stays with the body longer and eventually turns to fat...not good).

Apples are usually the most filling, but work with what you want.

Granola bars or sesame snacks are a good choice too, but be careful of the sugar content.

Dinner:

Try to eat dinner about 3-4 hours before you go to bed

and cook using olive oil, coconut oil and flax seed as they can help in digestion and in your overall mood.

Any of the following. Pick one from each class:

Class 1- chicken, tuna steak, beef steak, tofu (extra firm), salmon, or halibut.

Class 2- any combination of vegetables — usually best to stir fry in light vegetable oil, but do not overdo it on the sauce. Any of the vegetables mentioned above will be sufficient.

Class 3- rice or whole wheat pasta (usually brown rice is best) or sweet potatoes.

Add a small salad to that and you are good to go.

Snack at Night:

Be very careful here, as whatever you put in your body late at night has to digest quickly and easily. Keep it simple here, about 90 minutes before you go to bed (and of course it does not have to be followed so closely to the minute). For example, light yogurt or some other low-sugar, low-carbohydrate snack. You want to be able to fall asleep and not wake up at four o'clock in the morning, starving.

Now keep in mind with all of the above you will be getting hungry more often and you should be eating regularly to allow yourself to get hungry. However, the biggest thing here is creating options for yourself and not eating when you are starving. The proper food going into your system will allow you to maximize your workouts and help your mood and digestion throughout the day. Lastly, have nothing but water (or herbal tea as a hot beverage option) to drink. Aim for drinking 60 ounces of water per day. It will help fill you up, hydrate you, and do wonders for the gastrointestinal tract.

APPENDIX D
The Graduate School Application Process

So you have decided to pursue further education, go beyond the bachelor's degree, and tackle the master's, doctorate, medical, dental or law degree. Well, first things first. Coming in with a level head will make the first year much smoother for you. What is funny about graduate school is that the work involved is not overwhelmingly difficult; it is just that there is much more of it — a lot more! As an undergrad you may have had 10-page papers and now it is just 20-25 page papers. Instead of having periods of time where you are busy and then a lull, the lull part never comes in graduate school.

Many folks may come into a program worried that they do not match up or are not on par with their fellow students. It is like the big fish in a small pond theory: we may have been some of the best students in our undergraduate classes or graduate school, and then we come into a place where everyone is smart, successful, and motivated, and we feel average or inadequate. After struggling to get into graduate school and competing against others, you may immediately begin comparing yourself to the others in your class, and think you do not match up. You may have been so used to basing much of your own self-worth on academic performance that upon coming into graduate school you start feeling down early in the game.

However, in due time perspective will emerge that it is possible, and so as long as you are accepted into a program of your choice, you are as good as the other students. Do recall the person who finishes last in a medical school class is better-known as a doctor, and the average patient does not ask for a transcript of your grades when they seek medical attention.

Additionally, you may graduate with a law degree, or a master's in education or business administration and in fact never actually use it. Your career interests may change, but the bottom line is that you are capable, and it is possible to succeed. If you are thinking about applying, and you want the opportunity, do it! Do not hold back or limit yourself to areas of study and locations within the country. The graduate school experience does not define your life; it is just a part of it.

However, it is important that you know why you are applying. Is it because of family pressure, or social pressure to be a professional? You may not know where you want to apply, but before any application process begins it is important to know why; stay true to yourself and your ideals in that moment and do not live someone else's dream for them. Again, say to yourself: "This is my life, and I will make my choices."

Regardless of what you choose to do, if you go to graduate school know that you were accepted for good reasons, and that you deserve to be there. If you struggle, accept that you are struggling; know that others are too (even if they are too afraid or proud to say it). Know that less than a tenth of the people in the United States go on from college to graduate school, and far fewer pursue further degrees. It does not matter where you feel you rank, just that you get through it feeling you got all you could out of the experience. Stop the guilt and enjoy the experience!

20 Steps to Completing the
Graduate Application Process

1. **Buy this book and go through it:**

- Business Administration: *MBAMission Insider's guides series*
  By: mbaMission, from http://www.mbamission.com/store.php

- Dentistry: *The pre-dental guide: A guide for successfully getting into dental school*
  By: Joseph S. Kim

- Law: *How to get into the top law schools: The degree of difference series*
  By: Richard Montauk

- Medical School: *Medical School Admission Requirements (MSAR) 2012-2013: The most*

authoritative guide to U.S. and Canadian medical schools.
By: Association of American Medical Colleges

• Psychology: *Insider's guide to graduate programs in Clinical and Counseling Psychology 2012/2013 edition*
By: John C. Norcross, Michael A. Sayette & Tracy J. Mayne.

*Note: There are a variety of graduate schools and programs; if your field is not listed above, speak with a professor to find out what would be your best resource to purchase.

-1 week-

2. Make a list of all the possible schools you would consider attending (based on location, research preferences, and/or reputation). The list may be as long as thirty schools.

-1 weekend-

3. Meet with one or two faculty members from your program or peers who you feel could offer insight into the various schools.

-1 week-

4. Go through your list with the faculty you choose to meet. They will offer you honest opinions as to

which schools you can delete from your list and which schools you should definitely keep.

5. After meeting with faculty members, your list should be cut down to approximately ten schools. (*international students may apply to more)

-1 weekend-

6. Study and take the GRE or the required exam. If you have already done so, make sure your scores are high enough and that you have reached your desired score. If you need to take it again, that is okay!

-6 weeks-

7. Once you have your list finalized, go to the websites of each school and search their faculty lists to see which faculty members match your research interests.

-1 week-

8. E-mail/contact each of those faculty members stating that you feel your research interests match theirs, you would like to hear more about their research, and seek the opportunity to be a part of their research team. Make sure the email is no more than 200 words. Find at least three from each school to make sure you connect

with at least one.

-1 weekend-

9. Arrange a phone call or email correspondence with the professors from (8.).

-2 weeks-

10. Once you have connected with each faculty member from each school, then begin your statement of intent, incorporating the names of the faculty in your statement, if approproate. Have a friend and/or faculty member act as second reader to ensure your statement conveys everything you deem most necessary.

-2 weeks-

11. Go to each school's website and locate the addresses of where to send each document. **Note:** you may have to send your transcripts to a different address than the reference letters.

-1 weekend-

12. Construct a Word document that has a list of ALL the addresses in two columns. You should have two documents of addresses (i.e., for references and for transcripts). Also note which schools allow for reference letters to be sent online and others that need to be formally mailed.

Make sure you know how many copies of each transcript you will need for each school. You want to make the process of asking for reference letters and transcripts as easy as possible. Include your home address as one of the addresses so you know the transcripts were mailed. It is always a good thing to have an extra copy of your transcripts in your own file just in case they are needed immediately.

13. Make sure you send a packet or an e-mail with the proper links to each referee and the **list of addresses, one of your statements** so they are aware of your goals, and **a list of how you have connected with that person** (i.e., the courses you took with them, the research you were involved with) and **supplementary reference** letter forms for each school. **Note**: Many of the schools may have online reference forms or links to complete the reference letter, but to be on the safe side you may want to use the above instructions.

14. Finally, go to each website and fill out the graduate application online (each application takes approximately 35 minutes).

-1 week-

15. Once you have applied and received confirmation from the school, locate the GRE, MCAT, LSAT, or DAT institution codes and send all your scores to the required department or graduate

school. Make sure you have the **correct** code as sending each score costs *a lot*.

16. Attempt to have steps 1-15 completed by October 15-31 (or 6 weeks before the deadline), giving your references plenty of time to write your letters, the transcripts to reach the schools, and enough time to mail everything to them prior to Thanksgiving, for example. There are significant delays in the mail system after November 20th and the frequency of application materials sent to schools increases considerably after that.

17. Call the schools either right before or right after January 5th (or two weeks before the deadline) to ensure they have received all of your materials because there is a 100% chance they are missing something. Know that dates will vary between discipline and school; pay attention to the dates and adjust the above schedule accordingly.

18. The final step is the waiting game. Expect to hear back from schools around February or March. Invitations for interviews usually occurs beginning of February. Remember, the application process will not get you into school. The hope is that the application will grant you the interview — you are the one who gets you into the school with the right combination of your personality, aptitude, ability, experience, goals

and mindset.

19. Expenses – Be prepared to pay a lot of money. Each application involves the following expenses:
    - Application fee= $65.00
    - Transcript may cost up to $8.00
    - The transcript request(s) from some schools are free, but most are not. Just call the bursar's office and they will explain the process.
    - To mail items out to each school with a confirmation or tracking number (supplementary application forms, resume, statement of finances, writing samples , statement of intent, etc.) $10.00
    - GRE scores $15.00

    Total: **$100.00 USD**

20. <u>BREATHE</u> and prepare to live with uncertainty for a short time.

APPENDIX E
Mastering Your Interviews

1. BREATHE ... right this second. BREATHE. You know the breathing techniques/relaxation discussed earlier — do them for at least three minutes.

2. Take out that to-do list that you have, prioritize, and write down a time WHEN you will accomplish each task. No, you do not need to accomplish EVERYTHING... just the most important, to keep your focus days before the interview.

3. Stretch— whether that is 30 minutes of yoga or just 20 minutes of stretching exercises to loosen your muscles. You want to ensure you are at your most comfortable going in there — relieve that tension.

4. Set aside time to go through the material relevant to the interview WITHOUT overdoing it. Do NOT obsess about this. You cannot change the

job description, internship, or graduate school questions, you cannot change your experiences; you can change only your attitude and response to your current circumstances. Also be mindful of the questions you have for the interviewers.

5. Remember, they often do not care about what you did, as they know that already. They care about how what you did affected your life and essentially how you will fit with their world to make their lives easier. So, when thinking about your answers, think more about how the experience has created some effect on you and how the experience at the job/school/internship will help enhance that and simultaneously reach your goals and theirs.

6. You CANNOT control or guess what they will ask you, thinking about it/ obsessing about it will not help. So, know what they are looking for and be VERY familiar with how what they offer matches your current professional goals. Prove to them WHY and HOW you are a good fit. Ensuring that you maintain your focus. Everything else going on in life before or after will still be there, stay focused on the end goal: succeeding during the interview.

7. I know this job/internship/school acceptance is important to you AND it is not THE most important job/internship/school that will determine

whether you become the President of the United States. So, use the words: "It is a preference I get this job/internship/school acceptance and it is not a MUST." DO NOT place all the pressure on yourself; you are qualified and confident, and only you can tell yourself that.

8. If you think this job/internship/school acceptance is the ONLY thing you can do, you are placing an extensive amount of pressure on yourself...this is one opportunity that you ARE qualified for — now prove it!

9. Treat yourself — buy shoes, pick out your favorite outfit, go to a movie and DO NOT let the little things leading up to the interview become added stress...embrace it as something that will help you present yourself better.

10. EXERCISE: Engage in any type of exercise for 45 per day minutes throughout the week before, regardless of how tired you may be. Do this for yourself; exercise for you.

11. EATING: Do NOT rely on coffee or high sugars, or any caffeine for that matter. Be sure you are paying attention to your eating over the next few days: fiber, fruits, salads, and proteins. DRINK A LOT OF WATER. Keep the system in motion and/or do what is normal for you; do not change the routine.

12. BREATHE. Yes I said this again to remind you — breathe.

13. Start to visualize the interview. In the days leading up to the interview, imagine sitting in that room with the interviewer(s) and performing well. You have the passion and the skills to talk about it, whether you believe it or not. Remind yourself that you deserve to be there. YOU KNOW what you offer... prove it!

14. Remember, before the interview, go through your list of priorities and include a list of things for interview day (e.g., extra copies of your resume, pen, pad of paper with a folder, etc.). Make sure everything you need for the next day is prepared the night before so you can get ready blindfolded the morning of the interview.

15. There is no need for this interview to scare you, even if they ask you challenging questions. Step back and remind yourself of your experiences and how you articulate them will land you the job/internship/ school acceptance, the rest is in their hands. If you find yourself anxious at some point during the interview or just thinking about the unknown, step back and realize it is not a coincidence you landed the interview, you are not an impostor; you deserve to BE THERE!

16. No need to put all the pressure on you; put some on them. You are interviewing them just as

much, because for all we know you might not like the place at all, or how they handle their interviews. Ask them information about their world and what the working environment is like (e.g., collaborative teamwork is an important thing to me, what does that look like here within?)

17. DO NOT rush your answers. After each question is asked, take a second or two to think about it and to buy some time. It is tempting to just say whatever comes to mind first. Breathe before stepping forward into your answer; chances are it will help.

18. Know that each question is going to be only 2-3 minutes. If you make yourself think it is going to be like a lifetime, you are wrong. Each question is literally 2-3 minutes — no need to put more pressure on yourself than that. Realize 3 minutes, and that's it.

19. Use positive SELF-TALK. If you tell yourself you need to be worried and you need to be stressed, you will be. Just like in athletics, a little nervousness is okay. When you feel it starts to become more elevated, step back, breathe, relax various muscle groups, and reengage.

20. Keep your shoulders down!

REFERENCES

1. Self- talk

Vygotsky, L.S. (1962). *Thought and language.* Cambridge, MA: MIT Press. (Original work published 1934).

Piaget, J. (1965). *The language and thought of the child.* New York: Humanities Press.

Goodhart, D. E. (1986). The effects of positive and negative thinking on performance in an achievement situation. *Journal of Personality and Social Psychology, 51,* 117-124.

Van Raalte, J.L., & Brewer, B.W. (1995). Cork! The effects of positive and negative self-talk on dart throwing performance. *Journal of Sport Behavior, 18,* 50-58.

Hiebert, B., Uhlemann, M.R., Marshall, A., & Lee, D.Y.

(1998). The relationship between self-talk, anxiety, and counseling skills. *Canadian Journal of Counseling, 32*, 163-171.

Browne, F.R. (2005). Self-talk of group counselor: The research of Rex Stockton. *The Journal for Specialists in Group Work, 30*, 289-297.

Weinberg, R.S., & Gould, D. (2011). Foundations of Sport and exercise psychology (5th ed.), Champaign, Il: Human Kinetics.

Self-talk examples (1999, November). Retrieved on February 1, 2007 from http://www.kent.k12. wa.us/curriculum/assessment/testing_ABCs/ ModelPositiveSelfTalk.html

2. Relaxation

Jacobson, E. (1938). *Progressive Relaxation*. Chicago: University of Chicago Press.

Jacobson, E. (1970). *You must relax*. New York: McGraw-Hill Book Company.

Lehrer, P.M. (1996). Varieties of relaxation methods and their unique effects. *International Journal of Stress Management, 3*, 1-15.

Cheng, Y.L., Molassiotis, & Chang, A.M. (2003). The effect of progressive muscle relaxation training on anxiety and quality of life after stoma surgery in colorectal cancer patients. *Psycho-oncology, 12,* 254-266.

Matsumoto, M., & Smith, J.C. (2001). Progressive muscle relaxation, breathing exercises, and ABC relaxation theory. *Journal of Clinical Psychology, 57,* 1551-1557.

3. Imagery

Sackett, R.S. (1934). The influences of symbolic rehearsal upon the retention of a maze habit. *Journal of General Psychology, 13,* 113-128.

Schultz, J., & Luthe, W. (1959). *Autogenic training: A psychophysiologic approach to psychotherapy.* New York: Grune and Stratton.

Richardson, A. (1967a). Mental Practice: A review and discussion (Part 1). *Research Quarterly, 38,* 95-107.

Richardson, A. (1967b). Mental Practice: A review and discussion (Part 2). *Research Quarterly, 38,* 263-273.

Meichenbaum, D., & Turk, D. (1976). The cognitive behavioral management of anxiety, anger and pain. In P. Davidson (Ed.), *Behavioral management of anxiety, depression and pain.* New York: Brunner/ Mazel.

Worthington, E.L. Jr., & Shumate, M. (1981). Imagery and verbal counseling methods in stress inoculation for pain control. *Journal of Counseling Psychology,* *28,* 1-6.

Ford-Martin, P.A. (2004). *Gale encyclopedia of alternative medicine: Guided imagery.* Farmington Hills, MI: Thomson Gale.

Yoo, H.J., Ahn, S.H., Kim, S.B., Kim, W.K., & Han, O.S. (2005). Efficacy of progressive muscle relaxation training and guided imagery in reducing chemotherapy side effects in patients with breast cancer and in improving their quality of life. *Supportive Care in Cancer, 13,* 826-833.

4. Goal-setting

Bryan, J., & Locke, E. (1967). Goal setting as a means of increasing motivation. *Journal of Applied Psychology, 51,* 274-277.

Latham, G.P., & Yukl, G.A. (1975). A review of re- search on the application of goal setting in organizations. *Academy of Management Journal, 18,* 824-845.

Locke, E.A., Shaw, K.N., Saari, L.M., & Latham, G.P. (1981). Goal setting and task performance. *Psychological Bulletin, 90,* 125-152.

Erez, M. (1986). The congruence of goal-setting strategies with sociocultural values and its effect on performance. *Journal of Management, 12,* 585, 592.

Barrick, M., Mount, M., & Strauss, J. (1993). Conscientiousness and performance of sales representatives: Test of the mediating effects of goal setting. *Journal of Applied Psychology, 78,* 715-722.

Locke, E.A., & Latham, G.P. (2002). Building a practically useful theory of goal-setting and task motivation. *American Psychologist, 57,* 705-717.

MacLeod, A.K., Coates, E., & Hetherton, J. (2008). Increasing well-being through teaching goal-setting and planning skills: Results of a brief intervention. *Journal of Happiness Studies, 9,* 185-196.

5. Communication

Platt, J.H (1955). What do we mean "communication"? *The Journal of Communication, 5,* 21-26.

Berger, C.R., & Calabrese, R.J. (1975). Some explorations in initial interaction and beyond: Toward a developmental theory of interpersonal communication. *Human Communication Research, 1,* 99-112.

Berger, C. R. (1987). Communicating under uncertainty. In M.E. Roloff & G. R. Miller (Eds.), *Interpersonal processes: New directions in communication research* (p. 39-62). Newbury Park, C.A: Sage.

Berger, C.R. (2005). Interpersonal communication: Theoretical perspectives, future prospects. *Journal* of *Communication*, 55, 415-447.

6. Interpersonal Communication

Hargie, O., & Dickson, D. (2004). Skilled Interpersonal Communication: *Research, Theory and Practice*. Hove: Routledge.

Beebe, S.A., Beebe, S.J., & Redmond, M.V. (2007) *Interpersonal Communication: Relating to Others*. New York: Allyn & Bacon.

7. Happenstance

Krumboltz, J.D. (1979). A social learning theory of career decision making. In A.M. Mitchell, G.B. Jones & J.D. Krumboltz (Eds.), *Social Learning and career decision making*, (p.19-49), Cranston, R.I.: Carroll Press.

Krumboltz, J.D. (1996). A learning theory of career counseling. In M.L. Savickas & W.B. Walsh (Eds.), *Handbook of career counseling theory and practice*, (p.55-80), Palo Alto, CA: Consulting Psychologists Press.

Mitchell, K., Levin, A.S., & Krumboltz, J.D. (1999). Planned happenstance: Constructing unexpected career opportunities. *Journal of Counseling and Development, 77,* 115-124.

Krumboltz, J.D., & Levin, A.S (2004). *Luck Is No Accident:*

Making the Most of Happenstance in Your Life and Career. Atascadero, CA: Impact Publishers Inc.

Chien, J., Fischer, J.M., & Biller, E. (2006). Evaluating a Metacognitive and Planned Happenstance Career Training Course for Taiwanese College Students. *Journal of Employment Counseling, 43,* 146.

8. Nonverbal Communication

Darwin, C. R. (1872). *The expression of the emotions in man and animals.* London: John Murray.

Sherman, M.H., Ackerman, N.W., Sherman, S.N., & Mitchell, C. (1965). Non-verbal cues and reenactment of conflict in family therapy. *Family Process, 4,* 133-162.

Ekman, P., & Friesen, W. V. (1971). Constants across cultures in the face and emotion. *Journal of Personality and Social Psychology, 17,* 124-129.

Ekman, P., Friesen, W. V., O'Sullivan, M., Chan, A., Di- acoyanni-Tarlatzis, I., Heider, K., et al. (1987). Universals and cultural differences in the judgments of facial expressions of emotion. *Journal of Personality and Social Psychology, 53,* 712-717.

Russell, J. A. (1994). Is there universal recognition of emotion from facial expressions? A review of the cross-cultural studies. Psychological Bulletin, 115, 102-141.

Floyd, K., & Guerrero, L. K. (2006). *Nonverbal communication in close relationships*, Mahwah, NJ: Lawrence Erlbaum Associates.

Knapp, M. L., & Hall, J.A. (2007). *Nonverbal Communication in Human Interaction (5th ed.)*, Wadsworth: Thomas Learning.

9. Exercise

Morgan, W.P., Roberts, J.A., Brand, F.R., & Feinerman, A.D. (1970). Psychological effect of chronic physical activity. *Medicine and Science in Sports, 2,* 213-217.

Moses, J., Steptoe, A., Matthews, A., & Edwards, S. (1989). The effects of exercise training on mental well-being in the normal population: A controlled trial. *Psychometric Research, 33,* 47-61.

Anshel, M.H., Freedson, P., Hamill, J., Haywood, K., Horvat, M., & Plowman, S.A. (1991). *Dictionary of the sport and exercise sciences.* Champaign, Il: Human Kinetics Publishers.

Huang, Y., Macera, C. A., Blair, S. N., Brill, P. A., Kohl, H.W. III, & Kronenfeld, J. J (1998) . Physical fitness, physical activity, and functional limitation in adults aged 40 and older. *Medicine & Science in Sports & Exercise. 30,* 1430-1435.

Poupore, J. (1999). Lifestyle and structured exercise

programmes increased physical activity and improved cardiorespiratory fitness. *Evidence Based Nursing, 2,* 117-117.

Anshel, M.H., Reeves, L.H., & Roth, R.R. (2003). Concepts in fitness: A balanced approach to good health. Boston: Pearson Education.

Anshel, M.H. (2006). *Applied exercise psychology: A practitioner's guide to improving client health and fitness.* New York: Springer Publishing Company.

Durtine, J.L., Moore, G.E., Painter, P.L., & Roberts, S.D. (2009). ACSM's exercise management for persons with chronic diseases and disabilities. Champaign, II: Human Kinetics.

Gregorek, A., & Gregorek, J. (2009). The happy body: The simple science of nutrition, exercise, and relaxation. Woodside, CA: Jurania Press.

10. Attentional Control

Nideffer, R. (1976). Test of attentional and interpersonal style. *Journal of Personality and Social Psychology, 34,* 394-404.

Nideffer, R. (1981). *The ethics and practice of applied sport psychology.* Ithica, NY: Mouvement.

Folk, C.L., Remington, R.W., & Wright, J.H. (1994). The structure of attentional control: contingent attentional capture by apparent motion, abrupt on-set, and color. *Journal of Experimental Psychology: Human Perception and Performance, 20,* 317-329.

Teasdale, J.D., Segal, Z., & Williams, J.M.G. (1995). How does cognitive therapy prevent depressive relapse and why should attentional control (mindfulness) training help? *Behaviour Research and Therapy, 33,* 25-39.

Segal, Z.V., Williams, J.M., Teasdale, J.D., & Gemar, M. (1996). A cognitive science perspective on kindling and episode sensitization in recurrent affective disorder. *Psychological Medicine, 26,* 371-380.

11. Positive Reinforcement

Skinner, B. F. (1938). *The behavior of organisms.* New York: Appleton-Century-Crofts.

Skinner, B. F. (1956). A case history in scientific method. *American Psychologist, 11,* 21-33.

Turkat, I.D., & Adams, H.E. (1982). Covert positive rein-forcement and pain modification: A test of effica-cy and theory. *Journal of Psychosomatic Research, 26,* 191-201.

Forehand, R. (1986). Parental positive reinforcement with deviant children: Does it make a difference? *Child & Family Behavior Therapy, 8,* 19-25.

Hansen, T.L. (1990). A positive reinforcement program for controlling student absenteeism. *College Student Journal, 24,* 307-312.

Wilson, C., Boni, N., & Hogg, A. (1997). The effectiveness of task clarification, positive reinforcement and corrective feedback in changing courtesy among police staff. *Journal of Organizational Behavior Management, 17,* 65-99.

Chance, P. (2003). *Learning and Behavior.* (5th ed.) Toronto: Thomson-Wadsworth.

12. Music and Motivation

Schwartz, S. E., Fernhall, B., & Plowman, S. A. (1990). Effects of music on exercise performance. *Journal of Cardiopulmonary Rehabilitation 10,* 312-316.

Karageorghis, C. I., Terry, P. C., & Lane, A. M. (1999). Development and initial validation of an instrument to assess the motivational qualities of music in exercise and sport: The Brunel Music Rating Inventory. *Journal of Sports Sciences 17,* 713-724.

Karageorghis, C.I., Priest, D., Terry, P.C., Chatzisarantis, N.L.D., & Lane, A.M. (2006). Redesign and initial validation of an instrument to assess the motivational qualities of music in exercise: The Brunel Music Rating Inventory-2. *Journal of Sports Sciences, 24,* 899-909.

13. Eating Habits

Schwerin, H.S., Stanton, J.L. Smith, Riley,. A.M., Jr., & Brett, B.E. (1981). How has the quantity and quality of the American diet changed during the past decade? *Food Technology, 35,* 50-57.

Schwerin, H.S., Stanton, J.L. Smith, Riley, A.M., Jr., & Brett, B.E. (1982). Food, eating habits, and health: a further examination of the relationship between food eating patterns and nutritional health. *American Journal of Clinical Nutrition, 35,* 1319-1325.

Nestle, M. (2003) Increasing portion sizes in American diets: More calories, more obesity. *Journal of American Dietetic Association, 103,* 39-40.

National Heart, Lung, and Blood Institute (n.d.). Aim for a Healthy Weight, Patient and Public Education Materials. Retrieved on August 8, 2008 from www.nhlbi.nih.gov/health/public/heart/obesity/los e_wt/risk.htm

Zinczenko, D., & Goulding, M. (2011). Eat this not that!, no-diet diet: The world's easiest weight-loss plan! New York: Rodale Books.

14. Mindfulness

Kabat-Zinn, J. (1982). An out-patient program in Behavioral Medicine for chronic pain patients based on the practice of mindfulness meditation:

Theoretical considerations and preliminary results. *General Hospital Psychiatry, 4*, 33-47.

Kabat-Zinn, J., Lipworth, L., & Burney, R. (1985). The clinical use of mindfulness meditation for the self-regulation of chronic pain. *Journal of Behavioral Medicine, 8*, 163-190.

Kabat-Zinn, J., & Chapman-Waldrop, A. (1988). Compliance with an outpatient stress reduction program: rates and predictors of completion. *Journal of Behavioral Medicine, 11*, 333-352.

Gunaratana, B.H. (2002). *Mindfulness in Plain English, (Eds.)* Somerville, MA: Wisdom Publications.

15. Verbal Expression

Rogers, C. (1942). *Counseling and psychotherapy.* Boston: Houghton Mifflin.

Freud, S. (1949). *An outline of psychoanalysis.* New York: Norton.

Rogers, C. (1961). *On becoming a person.* Boston: Houghton, Mifflin.

Beck, A.T. (1963). Thinking and depression: Idiosyncratic content and cognitive distortions. *Archives of General Psychiatry, 9*, 324-333.

Perls, F. (1969). *Gestalt therapy verbatim.* Moah, UT:

Real People Press.

Lazarus, A.A. (1971). *Behavior therapy and beyond.* New York: McGraw-Hill.

Rogers, C. (1986). On the development of the person centered approach. *Person-Centered Review, 1,* 257-259.

Lambert, M. J., & Bergin, A. E. (1994a). The effectiveness of psychotherapy. In S. L. Garfield & A. E. Bergin (Eds.), *Handbook of psychotherapy and behavior change* (4th ed., p.143-189). New York: Wiley.

Sue, S., Zane, N., & Young, K. (1994b). Research on psychotherapy with culturally diverse populations. In A. E. Bergin & S. L. Garfield (Eds.), *Handbook of psychotherapy and behavior change* (4th ed., pp. 783–817). New York: Wiley.

Ellis, A. (1999). *How to make yourself happy and remarkably less disturbable.* San Luis Obispo, CA: Impact.

American Psychological Association Task Force on Evidence-Based Practice. (2006). Evidence-based practice in psychology. *American Psychologist, 61,* 271-285.

Sue, D.W., & Sue, D. (2008). *Counseling the Culturally Diverse: theory and practice,* (5th ed.). New York: John Wiley & Sons Inc.

16. Physical Expression

Parker, J., & Asher, S. (1987). Peer acceptance and ater personal adjustment: Are low acceptance children at risk? *Psychological Bulletin, 102,* 357-389.

Pepler, D., & Rubin, K. (1991). *The development and treatment of childhood aggression* (p.411-448). Hillsdale, NJ: Erlbaum.

Craig, W.M. (1998). The relationship among bullying, victimization, depression, anxiety, and aggression in elementary school children. *Personality and Individual Differences, 24,* 123-130.

Wolke, D., Woods, S., Bloomfield, L., & Karstadt, L. (2000). The association between direct and relational bullying and behaviour problems among primary school children. *Journal of Child Psychology and Psychiatry, 41,* 989-1002.

17. Written Expression

Pennebaker, J. W., Kiecolt-Glaser, J., & Glaser, R. (1988). Disclosure of traumas and immune function: Health implications for psychotherapy. *Journal of Consulting and Clinical Psychology, 56,* 239-245.

Donnelly, D.A., & Murray, E.J. (1991). Cognitive and emotional changes in written essays and therapy interviews. *Journal of Social and Clinical Psychology, 10,* 334-350.

L'Abate, L. (1992). *Programmed writing: A self- administered approach for interventions with individuals, couples, and families.* Pacific Grove, CA: Brooks/ Cole.

Smyth, J.M. (1998). Written emotional expression: Effect sizes, outcome types, and moderating variables. *Journal of Consulting and Clinical Psychology, 66,* 174-184.

18. Rational Emotive Behavior Therapy

Ellis, A. (1962). *Reason and emotion in psychotherapy.* Secaucus, N.J.: Citadel. Revised edition, Secaucus, N.J.: Carol Publishing Group, 1994.

Ellis, A., & Dryden, W. (1997). *The practice of rational emotive behavior therapy, (2nd ed.).* New York: Springer Publishing Company.

Ellis, A., & MacLaren, C. (2005). *Rational Emotive Behavior Therapy: A therapist's guide (2nd ed.).* Atascadero, CA: Impact Publishers.

Gregas, A.J. (2006). Applying multicultural rational emotive behavior therapy to multicultural classrooms. *Multicultural Learning and Teaching, 1,* 24-34.

19. Social Behavior

Homans, G.C. (1958). Social Behavior as Exchange. *American Journal of Sociology, 63,* 597-606.

Bagozzi, R.P. (1975). Social exchange in marketing. *Journal of the Academy of Marketing Science 3*, 314-327.

Kitchener, R.F. (1981). Piaget's Social Psychology. *Journal for the Theory of Social Behaviour, 11*, 253-277.

Triandis, H. C. (1989). The self and social behavior in differing cultural contexts. *Psychological Review, 96*, 506-520.

Turniansky, B., & Cwikel, J. (1996). Volunteering in a voluntary community: Kibbutz members and voluntarism. *Voluntas: International Journal of Voluntary and Nonprofit Organizations, 7*, 300-317.

Flynn, F.J., & Brockner, J. (2003). It's different to give than to receive: Predictors of givers' and receivers' reactions to favor exchange. *Journal of Applied Psychology, 88*, 1034-1045.

20. Social Network

Radcliffe-Brown, A.R. (1940). On social structure. *Journal of the Royal Anthropological Institute, 70*, 1-12.

White, H., Boorman, S., & Breiger, R. (1976). Social structure from multiple networks: I. Blockmodels of roles and positions. *American Journal of Sociology, 81*, 730-80.

Wasserman, S., & Faust, K. (1994). *Social Network Analysis: Methods and Applications*. Cambridge: Cambridge University Press.

Breiger, R. L. (2004). The Analysis of Social Networks. In M. Hardy & A. Bryman *Handbook of Data Analysis* (p. 505-526). London: Sage Publications.

Freeman, L. (2006). *The Development of Social Network Analysis*. Vancouver: Empirical Press.

21. Family and Culture

Sue, D.W., & Sue, D. (2008). *Counseling the Culturally Diverse: theory and practice, (5th ed.)*. New York: John Wiley & Sons Inc.

22. Parental Influences

Hoffman, M. L. (1960). Power assertion by the parent and its impact on the child. *Child Development, 31,* 129-143.

Hoffman, M. L. (1970). Moral development. In P. H. Mussen (ed.), *Carmichael's manual of child psychology* (Vol. 2, pp. 261–359). New York: Wiley.

Parsons, J., Adler, T., & Kaczala, C. (1982). Socialization of achievement attitudes and perceptions: Parental influences. *Child Development, 53,* 310-321.

Rohner, R. R. (1986). *The warmth dimension*. Newbury

Park, CA: Sage.

Baumrind, D. (1989). Rearing competent children. In W. Damon (Ed.) *Child development today and tomorrow* (p. 349–378). San Francisco: Jossey-Bass.

Rothbaum, F., & Weisz, J.R. (1994). Parental caregiving and child externalizing behavior in nonclinical samples: A meta-analysis. *Psychological Bulletin, 116*, 55-74.

Morrongiello, B.A., Corbett, M., & Bellissimo, A. (2008). Do as I say, not as I do: Family influences on children's safety and risk behaviors. *Health Psychology, 27*, 498-503.

23. Open Ended Questions

Johnson, W. R., Sieveking, N.A., & Clanton, E.S. (1974). Effects of alternative positioning of open-ended questions in multiple-choice questionnaires. *Journal of Applied Psychology, 59*, 776-778.

Myren, C. (1995). *Posing open ended questions in the primary classroom*. San Diego, CA: Teaching Resource Center.

Poorman, P.B. (2003). *Microskills and theoretical foundations for professional helpers*. Boston, MA: Allyn & Bacon.

Spörrle, M., Gerber-Braun, B., & Försterling, F. (2007).

The influence of response lines on response behavior in the context of open-question formats. *Swiss Journal of Psychology, 66,* 103–107.

24. Imaginary Play

Parten, M.B. (1932). Social participation among preschool children. *Journal of Abnormal and Social Psychology, 27,* 243-269.

Smilansky, S. (1968). *The effects of sociodramatic play on disadvantaged children: preschool children.* New York: Wiley.

Rubin, K.H., Watson, K.S., & Jambor, T.W. (1978). Free-play behaviors in preschool and kindergarten children. *Child Development, 49,* 534-536.

Ariel, S., & Sutton-Smith, B. (2002). *Children's imaginative play: A visit to wonderland.* Westport, CT: Praeger Publishers.

25. Social Anxiety

Markway, B.G, Carmin, C.N., Pollard, C.A., & Flynn, T. (1992). *Dying of embarrassment: Help for social anxiety and phobias.* Oakland, CA: New Harbinger Publications.

American Psychiatric Association. (2000). *Diagnostic and statistical manual of mental disorders,* 4th ed., Text Revision. Washington, DC: American

Psychiatric Association.

Antony, M.M., & Swinson, M.D. (2000). *The shyness and social anxiety workbook.* Oakland, CA: New Harbinger.

Chavira, D.A., & Stein, M.B. (2005). Childhood social anxiety disorder: From understanding to treatment. *Child and Adolescent Psychiatric Clinics of North America, 14,* 797-818.

Antony, M.M., & Swinson, M.D. (2008). *The shyness and social anxiety workbook*: Proven, step-by-step techniques for overcoming your fear (2nd ed.). Oakland, CA: New Harbinger.

26. Peer Pressure

Hochbaum, G.M. (1954). The relation between group members' self-confidence and their reactions to group pressures to uniformity. *American Sociological Review, 19,* 678-687.

Dielman, T.E., Campanelli, P.C., Shope, J.T., & Butchart, A.T. (1987). Susceptibility to peer pres- sure, self-esteem, and health locus of control as correlates of adolescent substance abuse. *Health Education & Behavior, 14,* 207-221.

Coggans, N., & McKellar, S. (1994). Drug use amongst peers: Peer pressure or peer preference? *Drugs: Education, Prevention & Policy, 1,* 15 – 26.

Orford, J., Krishnan, M., Balaam, M., Everitt, M., & Van Der Graaf, K. (2004). University student drinking: The role of motivational and social factors. *Drugs: Education, Prevention & Policy, 11*, 407-421.

27. Self-esteem

Rosenberg, M. (1965). *Society and the adolescent self-image*. Princeton, NJ: Princeton University Press.

Branden, N. (1969). *The psychology of self-esteem*. New York: Bantam.

Carlson, R. (1970). On the structure of self-esteem: Comments on Ziller's formulation. *Journal of Consulting and Clinical Psychology, 34*, 264-268.

Hill, S.E., & Buss, D.M. (2006a). The Evolution of Self-Esteem. In Michael Kernis, (ed.), *Self Esteem: Issues and Answers: A Sourcebook of Current Perspectives (p.*328-333). Psychology Press: New York.

Mruk, C. (2006b). *Self-Esteem research, theory, and practice: Toward a positive psychology of self- esteem* (3rd ed.). New York: Springer.

Buhlmann, U., Teachman, B.A., Gerbershagen, A., Kikul, J., & Rief, W. (2008). Implicit and explicit self- esteem and attractiveness beliefs among individuals with body dysmorphic disorder. *Cognitive Therapy and Research, 32*, 213-225.

28. Sexual Orientation

Kallmann, F.J. (1952). Comparative twin study on the genetic aspects of male homosexuality. *Journal of Nervous and Mental Disease, 115,* 283–97.

Hooker, E. (1957). The adjustment of the male overt homosexual. *Journal of Projective Techniques, 21,* 18-31.

Ellis, A., & Abarbanel, A. (1967). *Heterosexual relationships.* New York: Ace Publication Corporation.

Gonsiorek, J.C. (1982). Results of psychological testing on homosexual populations. *American Behavioral Scientist, 25,* 385-396.

Bohan, J.S., (1996). *Psychology and Sexual Orientation: Coming to Terms.* New York: Routledge.

Dorland, J.M., & Fischer, A.R. (2001a). Gay, lesbian, and bisexual individuals' perceptions: An analogue stuffy. *Counseling Psychologist, 29,* 532-547.

Russell, S.T., & Joyner, K. (2001b). Suicide attempts more likely among adolescents with same-sex sexual orientation. *American Journal of Public Health, 91,* 1276-1281.

Rosenberg, D. (2004, May 24). The 'Will & Grace.' *Newsweek,* 38-39.

Johnson, P. (2005). *Love, Heterosexuality and Society.* London: Routledge.

29. Dating

Kaplan, H. S., & Sager, C.L. (1971). Sexual patterns at different ages. *Medical Aspects of Human Sexuality, 1,* 10-23.

Parks, M. R., & Eggert, L. L. (1991). The role of social context in the dynamics of personal relationships. In W. Jones & D. Perlman (Eds.), *Advances in per- sonal relationships* (Vol. 2, pp. 1-34). London: Jessica Kingsley.

Harvey, J., Wenzel, A., & Sprecher, S. (2004). *Hand-book of sexuality in close relationships (Eds.),* Mahwah, NJ: Erlbaum Associates.

Molloy, J.T. (2004). *Why men marry some women and not others: The fascinating research that can land you the husband of your dreams.* New York: Warner Books.

Chapman, G. (2010). The five languages of love, men's Edition: The secret to love that lasts. Chicago, IL: Moody Publishers.

Chapman, G. (2012). The five languages of love: The secret to love that lasts. Chicago, IL: Moody Publishers.

30. Assertiveness

Smith, M. J. (1975). *When I say no, I feel guilty*. New York: Bantam Books.

Bower, S. A., & Bower, G. H. (1991). *Asserting Yourself: A Practical Guide for Positive Change* (2nd ed.). Reading, MA: Addison Wesley.

Alberti, R.E., & Emmons, M.L. (2008). *Your perfect right: A guide to assertive Living* (9th ed.). San Luis Obispo, CA: Impact Publishers.

31. Men and Emotions

Maiuro, R.D., Cahn, T.S., Vitaliano, P.P., Wagner, B.C., & Zegree, J.B. (1988). Anger, hostility, and depression in domestically violent versus generally assaultive men and nonviolent control subjects. *Journal of Consult- ing and Clinical Psychology, 56,* 17-23.

Pollack, W.S. (1998). Real boys: Rescuing our sons from the myths of masculinity. New York: Random House.

Cochran, S.V., & Rabinowitz, F.E. (2000). *Men and depression: Clinical and empirical perspectives*. San Diego, CA: Academic Press.

Mahalik, J.R., & Rochlen, A.B. (2006). Men's likely responses to clinical depression: What are they and do masculinity norms predict them? *Sex Roles, 55,* 659-667.

32. Self-Confidence

Haeger, F. (1931). Das Leistungsgefühl. / Self-confidence in work. *Psychotechnisches Zeitschrift, 6,* 148-152.

Mullins, C. J. (1963). Self-confidence as a response set. *Journal of Applied Psychology, 47,* 156-157.

Lenney, E. (1977). Women's self-confidence in achievement settings. *Psychological Bulletin, 84,* 1-13.

Jones, J. G., & Cale, A. (1989). Precompetition temporal patterning of anxiety and self-confidence in males and females. *Journal of Sport Behavior, 12,*183-195.

Stankov, L., & Crawford, J.D. (1997). Self-confidence and performance on tests of cognitive abilities. *Intelligence, 25,* 93-109.

Hanton, S., Mellalieu, S.D., & Hall, R. (2004). Self- confidence and anxiety interpretation: A qualitative investigation. *Psychology of Sport and Exer- cise, 5,* 477-495.

Miller, P.G. (2005). Scapegoating, self-confidence and risk comparison: The functionality of risk neutralisation and lay epidemiology by injecting drug users. *International Journal of Drug Policy, 16,* 246-253.

33. Substance Use Behavior

Kelleher, R.T., & Morse, W.H. (1968). Determinants of the specificity of behavioral effects of drugs In *Reviews of Physiology Biochemistry and Experimental Pharmacology, Vol. 60.* New York: Springer Berlin Heidelberg.

Baumeister, R.F. (1991). *Escaping the Self. Jackson,* TN: Basic Books.

Burnham, J.C. (1993). *Bad Habits: Drinking, Smoking, Taking Drugs, Gambling, Sexual Misbehavior, and Swearing in American History,* New York: University Press.

Lieber, C.S. (1994). Alcohol and the liver: 1994 update. *Gastroenterology, 106,* 1085-1105.

Ray, O., & Ksir, C. (1996). *Drugs, society, and human behavior (7th ed.).* St. Louis, MO: Mosby-Year Book Inc.

Benshoff, J.J., & Janikowski, T.P. (2000). *The rehabilitation model of substance abuse counseling.* Belmont, CA: Wadsworth.

Rorer, K. (2002, March 1). Ketamine: An Escape From Reality. Retrieved on August 1, 2008 from http://serendip.brynmawr.edu/bb/neuro/neuro02/web1/krorer.html#1

Brandt, A.M. (2007). *The Cigarette Century; The rise and deadly persistence of the product that defined America*, New York: Basic Books.

34. Aggressive Communication

Norton, R. W. (1978). Foundation of a communicator style construct. *Human Communication Research, 4*, 99-112.

Gorden, W. I., & Infante, D. A. (1987). Employee rights: Context, argumentativeness, verbal aggressiveness, and career satisfaction. In C. A. B. Osigweh (Ed.), *Communicating employee responsibilities and rights* (p.149-163). Westport, CT: Quorum.

Bayer, C. L., & Cegala, D. J. (1992). Trait verbal aggressiveness and argumentativeness: Relations with parenting style. *Western Journal of Communication, 56*, 301-310.

Kassing, J. W., & Avtgis, T. A. (1999). Examining the relationship between organizational dissent and aggressive communication. *Management Communication Quarterly, 13*, 100-115.

Rancer, A. S., & Avtgis, T. A. (2006). *Argumentative and aggressive communication*. Thousand Oaks, CA: Sage.

Rancer, A.S., & Nicotera, A.M. (2007). Aggressive Communication. In B.B. Whaley, & W. Samter, (Eds).

Explaining communication: Contemporary theories and exemplars. (pp. 129-147). Mahwah, NJ: Lawrence Erlbaum Associates Publishers.

35. Passive Communication

Sherman, R. (1999, January). Understanding your communication style. Retrieved on August 31, 2008 from http://www.au.af.mil/au/awc/awcgate/sba/comm_style.htm

Ryan, E.B., Kennaley, D.E., Pratt, M.W., & Shumovich, M.A. (2000). Evaluations by staff, residents, and community seniors of patronizing speech in the nursing home: Impact of passive, assertive, or humorous responses. *Psychology & Aging, 15,* 272-285.

Key to Success: How to Understand Four Communication Styles (2005). Retrieved on August 1, 2008 from http://www.afroarticles.com/article- dashboard/ Article/Key-to-Success—How-to- Understand-Four-Communication-Styles/86711

36. Chinese Proverb

Inspirational words of wisdom (2008, August) One moment of patience may ward off great disaster. One moment of impatience may ruin a whole life." retrieved on March 10, 2007. http://64.233.167.104/search?q=cache:YjD9d_c69 UkJ: www.wow4u.com/ pa- tience/index.html+%22One+moment+of+patience

...%22&hl=en&ct=clnk&cd=3&gl=us

37. The Paradox of Our Age

Moorehead, B. (1995). The Paradox of age. In *Words Aptly Spoken*, Redmond, WA: Overlake Christian Bookstore.